simply well

simply well

CHOICES FOR A HEALTHY LIFE

by John W. Travis, MD, and Regina Sara Ryan

Ten Speed Press
Berkeley / Toronto

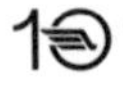 Ten Speed Press
Box 7123
Berkeley, California 94707
www.tenspeed.com

Distributed in Australia by Simon & Schuster Australia, in Canada by Ten Speed Press Canada, in New Zealand by Southern Publishers Group, in South Africa by Real Books, in Southeast Asia by Berkeley Books, and in the United Kingdom and Europe by Airlift Book Company.

Cover design by Catherine Jacobes
Book design by Betsy Stromberg
Illustrations on pages 9 and 15 by Ellen Sasaki

Some of the material in this book originally appeared in *Wellness: Small Changes You Can Use to Make a Big Difference* by Regina Sara Ryan and John W. Travis, MD, published in 1991 by Ten Speed Press.

Library of Congress Cataloging-in-Publication Data

Travis, John W.
Simply well : choices for a healthy life / by John W. Travis
and Regina Sara Ryan. - [10th anniversary ed.].
p. cm.
Rev. ed. Of: Wellness / Regina Sara Ryan. c1991.
Includes index.
ISBN 1-58008-292-0
1. Health. I. Ryan, Regina Sara.
II. Ryan, Regina Sara. Wellness. III. Title.
RA776 .R93 2001
613-dc21
2001027173

Printed in Canada
First printing, 2001

1 2 3 4 5 6 7 8 9 10 — 05 04 03 02 01

Disclaimer: It is not the intent of the authors to diagnose or prescribe, nor is it the purpose of this book to replace the services of a health professional. This material is intended for educational purposes only. It is advisable to seek the advice of a licensed, professional health-care provider for any condition that may require medical or psychological attention.

acknowledgments

With deepest appreciation to my husband, Jere Pramuk, who supports and celebrates my life. To John for sharing the labor and keeping the vision. Thanks to Kirsty Melville and Julie Bennett, our publisher and our editor, for help and encouragement in producing this millennium edition.

—RSR

To my daughters, Hannelore Travis Barnes and Siena Travis Callander, and my wife, Meryn Callander, who keep me ever learning more about myself and wellness.

—JWT

dedication

*

For Lee Khépá Baul

For Meryn, Siena, and Hannelore

contents

Introduction

*

Simplicity is an enormously compelling notion. Today, especially in the domains of health, we are literally deluged with data about what to eat, what supplements to take, how to best exercise, and how to express our feelings. The more options we have, whether in health or in other areas of life, the more we look for and need simple, clear maps that guide us through the labyrinth of information, technology, and goods and services that surround us. *Simply Well* is just such a guidebook—a bare-bones, commonsense and enjoyable approach to health of body, mind, and spirit, based on a foundation of education, self-awareness, and self-responsibility.

When we are ill, or looking to make a change in lifestyle to support our health, help is certainly appreciated, but an overload of input can actually become a burden, compounding confusion and raising doubts, convincing us that things are much more difficult than they are. Even after we have set a reasonable course for ourselves, we may hear that certain "experts" have found the very strategies we are using to be worthless or even damaging. To make matters worse, well-meaning friends and family members have unending opinions about and prescriptions for our health. Imagine having a chest cold that you are handling quite well with rest and liquids. At a meeting with a group of friends, you cough a few times and are immediately offered a string of unsolicited advice about what you could (and in fact should) do about it; advice that ranges from a formula for making garlic and walnut tea to seeing a doctor before the cold turns into pneumonia. Sound familiar? In times like these, we need the simple self-confidence that comes from knowing our body and trusting our experience in what works best for us. Building that confidence by education and self-awareness is what *Simply Well* is all about.

Far from simple, the human body is a miracle of complexity. Its ability to adjust to a wide range and quality of input and to enact wondrous transformations is nothing short of miraculous. Our bodies magically transform food into muscle and blood, ovum and sperm into child, breath and voice into communication. If we had to consciously monitor each of these functions, we would be a sorry species. Some of us forget to brush our teeth; imagine if we had to monitor every breath!

While our bodies may be complex in their functioning, good health is really quite simple. Basic healthiness is the organism's standard condition, as systems generally seek balance (or homeostasis) and will maintain this condition unless deprived or interfered with. Generally speaking, good health is our birthright. The human task is to be a responsible caretaker of the inherent wisdom that already governs the body. Give your body the raw materials of fresh food, water, and air, move it vigorously, supply it with life-affirming stimulation, encourage it to establish caring relationships with others, and it will generally work like a charm. When temporarily weakened or ill, your body can draw on two billion years of active, balance-seeking instinctive heritage to propel it back on course. The choices recommended in this book all favor trusting and responding to your body's natural wisdom and inclinations to guide you toward good health and wellness.

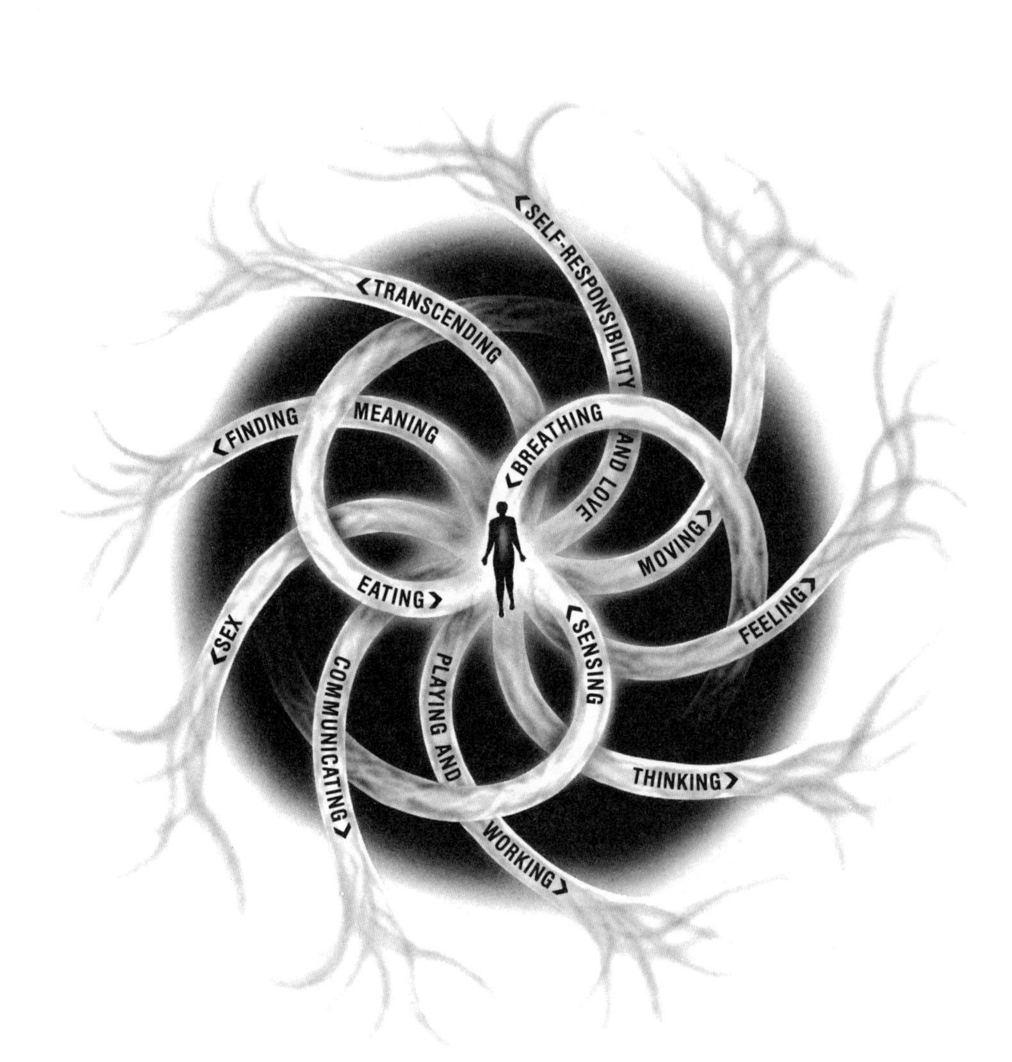

***The Wellness Energy System** has twelve components—three are the major sources of energy input: eating, breathing, and sensing; and nine are forms of energy output: self-responsibility and love, moving, feeling, communicating, thinking, sex, working and playing, finding meaning, and transcending.*

The Wellness Energy System *

Everything is energy—including the paper in your hands and the thoughts you are now thinking as you read this. Your body/mind/spirit is a sophisticated *energy transformation system.*

You take in energy from all the sources around you—from such tangible inputs as air, food, heat, light, sound, and physical touch, and from less tangible emotional and spiritual inputs as attention, care, love, enthusiasm, and extrasensory data.

You organize and transform that energy—some for internal housekeeping (such as digestion, circulation, and neural activity), some for tissue repair, and some to generate emotions and thinking processes, including spiritual insights and transcendent states of consciousness.

You return some energy to the environment around you—for instance, as heat or carbon dioxide. You also return energy through communication and physical work, and through your expression of emotions and creativity.

The Wellness Energy System is our alternative to the usual piecemeal way of looking at health. We offer an integrated overview of all human life functions, seeing them as various forms of energy. The harmonious balancing of these life functions results in good health and wellbeing.

Illness and Energy

When the flow of energy in your system is balanced and smooth, you feel good. When there is interference

* Adapted from Travis, J., and Ryan, R., *Wellness Workbook* (Ten Speed Press, 1981, 1988). First developed by John Travis in 1976, the Wellness Energy System is the theoretical framework for both this book and the *Wellness Workbook.*

in the flow, illness is often the result. Interference can occur at any point. It could be due to:

* low quality or insufficient input energy—such as polluted air or a poorly balanced diet
* an insufficient or weak transformer—such as a damaged heart or an overweight body
* blockages to output energy—such as the inability to express emotions or no one with whom to communicate

As a human being you are an energy transformer, connected with the whole universe. The condition of each of your life processes, including the illness and wellness processes, depends on how you manage energy.

The challenge of being well, then, is the challenge of maximizing the efficiency of your energy transformation system.

Although our body essentially knows what it needs, both in quantity and quality, we often give it much more or much less. We have been trained over a lifetime to listen to the demands of our mind rather than the pleas of our body; we seek immediate comfort rather than allowing the time and supplying the resources that will help our body heal or realign itself. The media has convinced us that we need more, more, more; bigger, fancier, and better; or somehow different. We don't. Regardless of what we have been led to believe, we do not *need* a whole shelf full of vitamins, minerals, and other assorted supplements to be healthier (although most people's diets do require *some* supplementation of minerals and vitamins). We do not need an expensive array of exercise equipment or a wardrobe of workout clothes and special shoes. We do not need a membership in a gym or health club, even though these facilities can be beneficial. We do not need a personal trainer or a live-in masseuse and beautician. Nor do we need a degree in nutrition and microbiology to keep ourselves well. As this book will illustrate, good health is as simple as choosing to take a full, energizing, and relaxing breath, right now. Inhale . . . exhale . . . ahhh.

To be "simply well" is to honor the simple basics of life, to appreciate the raw essentials of what it means to be human, to acknowledge honestly what we must do to foster who we *really* are, with a minimum of overlays. When we aren't lost in the "stuff" of health (or anything else), we can listen to ourselves (body, mind, and soul are "speaking" to us all the time) about what we genuinely want and need. We can "listen" to the many cues and clues that our surroundings have for us (through the words of other people, through the way events turn out, through what we see or hear) without being overwhelmed; taking and using what is worthwhile to us, while discarding the rest without strings attached. Furthermore, as we get back in touch with ourselves in the simple and basic ways that this book suggests, we find that we are not so different from others. Recognizing our interdependence, we set the stage for true compassion and genuine service to others. We are encouraged, when we rest in simple awareness and simple wellbeing, to view birth, growth, and creativity, along with weakness, illness, and death, as normal aspects of life's unfolding mystery.

Simply Well is structured around thirty-two life-affirming topics, each one inviting you to make healthier choices for yourself. The choices are simple, but not all easy, and will require thought and effort. If you've spent twenty, forty, or sixty years establishing a group of habits, any one of which is draining your lifeforce, it will likely take loving yet firm and consistent effort to turn yourself around. Use this book to begin or continue your exploration into the realm of healthier choices. Most of our "choices" in the area of health are better termed "reactions" since they are propelled by practices passed to us from our parents and family members, media hype, genetic heritage, and many other factors that influence us—generally unconsciously. *Simply Well* encourages greater self-awareness or consciousness—helping us break through the usual mechanical response to life. Breaking through, we catch a glimpse of how much more simple, spontaneous, and enjoyable life can be.

The Iceberg Model of Health and Disease *

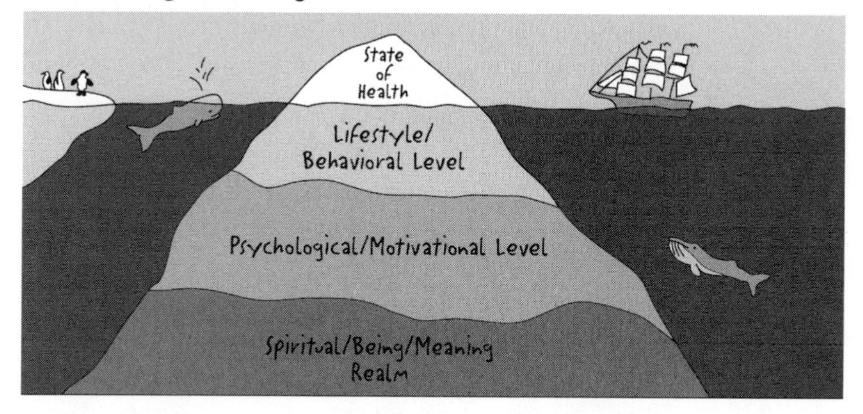

Icebergs reveal only about one-tenth of their mass above the water. The remaining nine-tenths are submerged. This is why they are such a nightmare in navigation, and why they make such an appropriate metaphor in considering your state of wellness.

Your current state of health—be it one of disease or of vitality—is just like the tip of the iceberg. This is

* Adapted from Travis, J., and Ryan, R., *Wellness Workbook* (Ten Speed Press, 1981, 1988).

the apparent part, what shows. If you don't like it, you can attempt to change it, do things to it, chisel away at an unwanted condition. But whenever you knock some off, like the iceberg, more of the same comes up to take its place.

To discern everything that creates and supports your current state of health, you have to look below the surface. The first level you'll encounter is the Lifestyle/Behavioral Level—what you eat, how you use and exercise your body, how you relax and let go of stress, and how you safeguard yourself from the hazards around you.

Many of us follow lifestyles that we know are destructive, both to our own wellbeing and to that of our planet. Yet we may feel powerless to change them. To understand why, we must look still deeper, to the Psychological/Motivational Level. Here we find what leads us to a certain way of life. We can learn, for example, what payoffs we get from being overweight, smoking, or driving recklessly, or from eating well, being considerate of others, and getting regular exercise.

Your culture's norms powerfully affect your daily thoughts and habits—often in subtle or insidious ways. Cultural norms, combined with the long-lasting effects of dysfunctional childhood experiences (e.g., growing up in a family where emotions were suppressed or inappropriately expressed), serve to keep people on automatic, repeating self-destructive patterns for a lifetime. You can break out of these cycles by reevaluating the environment you create around you—friends, workplace, and home—and making appropriate changes.

Cultural Norms and Wellness

Cultural norms are the beliefs and values generally accepted by a population. Your culture's norms guide everything from your sexual behavior to the career path you choose to what you eat for breakfast. Cultural norms either encourage or undermine health and wellness. In the past twenty years, the cultural norms for running and other forms of solitary exercise have changed dramatically, as has cultural acceptance of smoking, especially in public places.

Researchers have found that cultural norms usually lag years behind what the majority of people privately think or practice. This lowest common denominator effect serves to maintain common behaviors that encompass the total population even if most people actually think they are outmoded and inadequate.

We shape the culture in our image, just as it shapes us.

STARHAWK,
Dreaming the Dark

Cultural norms change when enough individuals adopt a new attitude or behavior within their own lifestyles. It is important, therefore, not to underestimate the power of one person to make a difference. Just as your personal wellness process can begin with small changes in your lifestyle, so too can these small changes help to alter cultural norms.

Exploring below the Psychological/Motivational Level, we encounter the Spiritual/Being/Meaning Level. This could also be called the transpersonal, philosophical, or metaphysical level. Actually, we prefer to call it a realm rather than a level because it has no clear boundaries. This realm includes the mystical and the mysterious, everything in the unconscious mind, and concerns issues such as your reason for being, the real meaning of your life, and your place in the universe. How you address these questions and the answers you choose underlie and permeate all of the layers above. Ultimately, this realm determines whether the tip of the iceberg, representing your state of health, is one of disease or wellness.

Your choices are matters of life and death. The accumulated effect of small choices you make every day creates a basic orientation toward vibrant wellness in one direction, illness and unconscious life in the other.

It's your call. This book can help you take charge of your life and health and tap your inner resources in a practical and effective way.

This book is about wellness, a subject that we have written about, taught, and lived with for over sixty years of combined experience. We have discovered that wellness is not a state you achieve once and for all. There is no end point in wellness, and as with every other process in life, it will have its highs and lows. You will make strides and live the positive results of those advances—in energy, strength, and vitality in general. You will also have periods when you need to rest, evaluate, recuperate, or change direction. What works today may not work tomorrow. Truly, life is never static and neither is our experience of wellness. What you are starting here, or continuing, is a way of life, not a series of prescriptions.

Nor is wellness a limited or exclusive concept. Although many people associate it only with fitness, nutrition, or stress reduction, it is much more. Wellness is a way of life that takes people into realms far beyond treatment or therapy—toward self-responsibility and self-empowerment. If you are ill, the wellness approach works alongside any forms of treatment you may be undertaking with your doctor or health professional,

The Illness/Wellness Continuum

Moving from the center to the left shows a progressively worsening state of health. Moving to the right from center indicates increasing levels of health and wellbeing. The Treatment Model (drugs, herbs, surgery, psychotherapy, and so on) can only bring you to the neutral point, alleviating the symptoms of disease. The Wellness Model, which can be used at any point on the continuum, helps you move toward higher levels of wellness. The Wellness Model is not intended to replace the Treatment Model, but to work in harmony with it. If you are ill, treatment is important, but don't stop at the neutral point. Use the Wellness Model to move toward high-level wellness.

encouraging you to become an active participant in the healing process instead of a passive recipient.

We have divided the book into four main sections, loosely structured to guide you from the basics to more advanced considerations within the field of wellness. Move at whatever pace feels right to you.

PART I, STARTING POINTS, will orient you for the journey ahead by helping you bring what you already know into conscious awareness and by encouraging you to set goals for the results you want to achieve. This section will supply you with a handful of essential tools you can use along the way, such as ways to handle stress and strong emotions. You will learn the art of inhabiting your body, developing self-awareness and self-appreciation so you can become your own best friend, teacher, and healer.

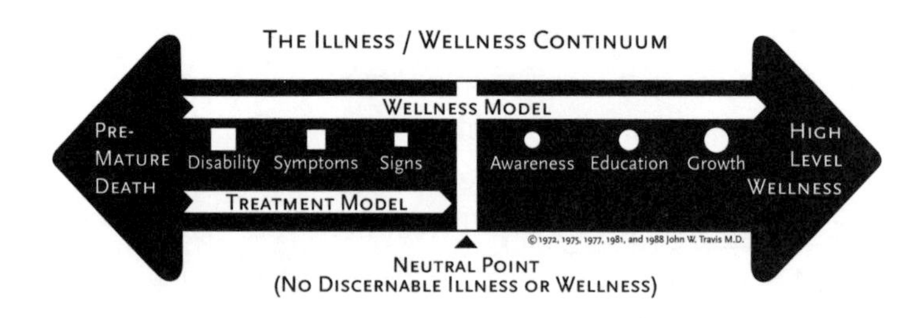

PART II is called LOOSENING UP and is designed to help you gently and gradually stretch into your new choice for a wellness lifestyle. You will be invited and encouraged to lighten up through laughter, therapeutic touch, meditation, and other soft exercises. Good health need not be a grim proposition, but rather can be nurtured and maintained with simple and enjoyable approaches.

In PART III, we get down to the business of TAKING ACTION. By now you will be limbered up and ready to take initiative in areas that require a bit more energy or a stronger commitment—like starting an exercise program, restructuring your relationship to food, building a support system, or changing your job. Not everything in this section will be useful to everyone, but there is surely something for everybody.

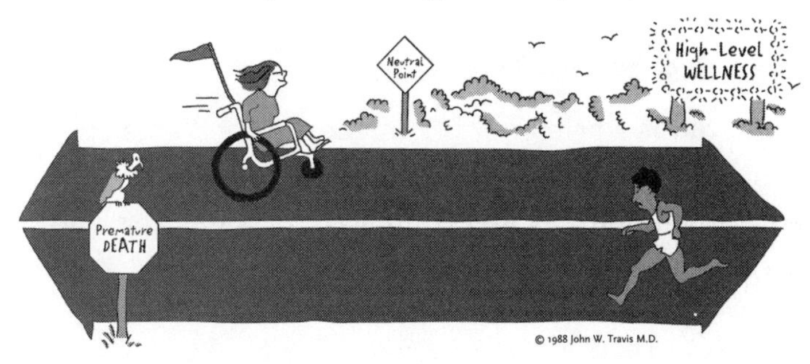

THE ILLNESS/WELLNESS CONTINUUM REVISITED

The Illness/Wellness Continuum Revisited

Wellness is your right and privilege regardless of your current state of health or illness. There is no prerequisite other than your free choice. A "well" being is not necessarily a strong, brave, successful, young, or even illness-free person. You can pursue wellness even if you are physically disabled, aged, scared in the face of challenge, in pain, imperfect. Sound familiar? The direction in which you are headed is what's important. Regardless of where you are on the Illness/Wellness Continuum, you can make some small change, right now, that will orient you toward higher levels of wellness, and this book will show you how.

PART IV is called ONE STEP BEYOND. It provides a more complete understanding of wellbeing. Have you ever considered the powerful effects of sound or silence in structuring a healthy environment, the healing power of forgiveness, or the value of living with death as a friend and advisor? This section presents you with possibilities for enhancing your spiritual life. Because the journey to wellness is an integrated process, you'll notice cross-references in the margins that lead you from one chapter to other chapters. If a subject we're discussing in Chapter 3 is discussed in more detail or in a slightly different manner in Chapters 7, 10, and 23, we want you to be able to find those discussions easily. Still want more? For those who wish to pursue this subject of wellness further, the resources section will give you ways to find more in-depth information.

How Best to Use This Book

This book is a primer. It is a memory jogger, an inspiration generator, and a referral guide filled with simple actions to improve your health and wellbeing. Use it as such and you will be using it to full advantage. Here are a few suggestions to keep in mind:

* BEGIN AT THE BEGINNING. If wellness is new to you, we suggest that you work your way through the book sequentially to get the benefit of building from the ground up. However, the information and suggestions presented in each chapter stand alone, and you can jump in anywhere. Decide how you learn best and proceed that way. If you have a particular need or interest, check the table of contents to find the areas that address it.

* BE ACTIVE. This is a mini-workbook, not a novel to get lost in. Stay active by doing the exercises. Think about your choices. Challenge and question whether our suggestions are congruent with your own experience. Mark what you want to remember or study further.

* ASK FOR HELP. Create a wellness partnership or a support system for yourself as you work through this book. Or better yet, share the journey with a friend who will engage in the process along with you. Even if you are sure of yourself, or thoroughly trained in some health system, it helps to have someone else with whom to share the healing journey—someone to talk to, someone to give you feedback or a reality check once in a while, someone to keep you encouraged, and above all, someone to care about you. So whether it is a good

There are two ways of being happy—we may either diminish our wants or augment our means—either will do—the result is the same; and it is for each to decide and do that which happens to appeal the most to them. If you are idle, or sick, or poor, however hard it may be to diminish your wants, it will be harder to augment your means. If you are active and prosperous, or young, or in good health, it may be easier for you to augment your means than to diminish your wants. But if you are wise you will do both at the same time, young or old, rich or poor, sick or well; and if you are very wise, you will do both in such a way as to augment the general happiness of society.

BENJAMIN FRANKLIN

friend or family member, a helping professional, or a support group, let yourself lean on someone else once in a while.

Think about who in your life currently supports you. Who can you rely on for comfort? For clarification or information? For confrontation when they observe you going off track? Who can you rely on for inspiration? Think about personal resources, like your friend down the block who can always be called in an emergency, or an acquaintance who works in a social service agency. Many times people fail to ask for the help they need because they have either forgotten how many resources they actually have or are hesitant to call on them. Make a list.

* EXPECT LOTS OF QUESTIONS. This book is not about absolute prescriptions, specific diets, or regimented exercise programs, even though all of these things are considered. We believe wellness has much more to do with developing self-awareness—learning to trust your own internal guidance system through the information that your body is giving you. This is the key to creating your own vibrant life in your own way. That may mean asking some serious questions—honest questions that guide you in discovering honest answers about yourself. These questions usually lead you to other questions,

motivating further awareness, education, and growth. Our goal is to raise more questions than we answer and to help you generate and refine your questions. Learning to live with ambiguity is also part of wellness.

* START A WELLNESS JOURNAL OR DIARY. Writing regularly about what you are learning and remembering about your life and health is a powerful tool for continued motivation. Our students and workshop participants are generally surprised at how much they know about themselves once they start putting their thoughts and feelings on paper. Writing helps to integrate separate aspects of your wellness into a whole picture. As you put your practices and experiences into words, you are using another modality, which will strengthen their impact on your life. Reading back over the changes that you have made and continue to make will help you chart your progress, giving you additional encouragement to keep going.

You don't need to limit your journal keeping to formal writing. Try writing poetry or drawing pictures to express your experiences.

* SET SHORT-TERM GOALS FOR YOURSELF. Frequently evaluate your learning and reward yourself in healthy ways for your progress. Be open to modifying

See Chapter 5: Discover What You Already Know (page 46) and Chapter 8: Set Goals for the Changes You Want to Make (page 61) for more information on setting goals.

See Chapter 28: Heal with Compassion (page 187) for more information on forgiveness.

your goals as necessary. As you maintain momentum in the direction of your original intention, something might intervene and start you on another course that is even more desirable than your initial one.

Take it easy on yourself. Give yourself the benefit of a friendly attitude or compassionate acceptance as you encounter areas that need a lot of work. Avoid compounding ill health or disease by burdening yourself with guilt about what you are doing or not doing. Make mistakes and keep on going. You may start with a burst of energy but be unable to maintain that pace. Make each day a new beginning. Simply renew your intentions and practice forgiveness for what you haven't done.

Important: If, as you are working with this book, you find that your problems seem bigger than you, it is essential that you get help. Don't wait. Seek out a helping professional or a support group that has experience with your particular problem—whether that is alcoholism, an eating disorder, depression, cancer, AIDS, or any other condition.

* Refer to the resources. At the end of the book we have suggested additional books you might read to expand your understanding of wellness. We go into greater depth regarding most of the small steps covered in this book in our *Wellness Workbook* (Ten Speed Press, 1981, 1988). The *Wellness Workbook* is available at bookstores or by mail.

Part I
starting points

*

A GOOD BEGINNING IS SIMPLE: You recall what you already know; you set a goal for yourself; you take a step, now, to move you in the direction of that goal.

Start here. Part I contains eight areas that will orient your initial steps toward wellness and will provide you with foundation skills that will prove useful all along the way. Welcome to the journey to wellness.

USE PART I TO:

* consider simplifying your life
* honor the innate wisdom of your body
* breathe better to feel better
* appreciate the role of emotions in health
* discover what you already know about wellbeing
* "program" yourself for health

* connect to nature for healing and a healthier perspective
* set goals for your wellness journey

1 Become a Beginner—Simplify

I like to live always at the beginnings of life. . . . I am by nature always beginning. . . .

Anaïs Nin

Becoming well in body and mind and spirit is our focus in this book. Ageless wisdom teaches that only when you are experiencing life simply, and celebrating its ordinariness, are you living in harmony. In contemporary times, the Zen master and scholar Suzuki Roshi has termed this approach to life the "beginner's mind."

Wellness is not a matter of accumulating something—like more data or more special programs. Rather, wellness is realized by being present and unburdening yourself of all that prevents a natural state of basic healthiness. To be well is to become more simple. Here are a few suggestions to get you thinking and moving like a beginner.

Begin to Be a Beginner

* Simplify your stuff. How can you expect newness, freshness, and surprises if every square inch of space in your home and every corner of your mind is filled with

"stuff"? It is beneficial to leave room around you for something mysterious to take place in life. Consider how your "stuff" may be a burden or may keep you trapped because it identifies you with the past and with a limited definition of who you are. Consider whether or not you would like to make a change here. Try giving a bunch of stuff away and learn what happens.

* SIMPLIFY YOUR DIET. How natural, fresh, and true to their original color are the foods you currently eat? Foods that are cooked simply or eaten raw tend to supply many more nutrients than those that are "worked over" in a variety of ways. Refining your diet in this way can have profound effects on the quality of your entire life.

* SIMPLIFY YOUR LIFE. Look carefully at all the ways in which your energy is being used, and note especially where and how it is being drained away. What might happen if you simply said yes when you meant yes and no when you meant no?

Take time to rest your mind. Use nature as a source of healing and meditation or prayer as a daily practice for keeping attuned to what is important. When the big picture is kept in the forefront, the little things just fall into line.

Consult Chapter 12: Drink More Water—And Other Healthy Uses of H_2O (page 88), Chapter 16: Develop Personal Nutritional Awareness (page 119), Chapter 17: Learn Ten Basics about Food (page 125), and Chapter 27: Create a Bigger Picture of Health (page 181) for ways to create a more healthy diet.

See Chapter 21: Just Say No (page 148) for help in saying what you mean.

The great majority of us are required to live a life of constant systematic duplicity. Your health is bound to be affected if, day after day, you say the opposite of what you feel, if you grovel before what you dislike and rejoice at what brings you nothing but misfortune. Our nervous system isn't just a fiction; it's a part of our physical body, and our soul exists in space and is inside us, like the teeth in our mouth. It can't be forever violated with impunity.

BORIS PASTERNAK

See your loved ones as brand-new every day. After living with people for years, adults or children, it is easy to develop the notion that you really know them. And in some ways you do. Yet it is a trap to always anticipate their reactions to certain things. Doing that almost assures that you will get just what you have expected. Acknowledge that human beings are much more complex and mysterious than that. There are always surprises to be uncovered, always new depths of appreciation that can be explored. Allowing someone else to be brand-new may start with pretending or imagining that you are meeting them again, for the very first time. It works.

Watch your language and your thoughts. Expressions like "I'm too old for that . . ." should be red flags, signaling you to become a beginner again.

Turn problems upside down, especially health problems. Instead of assuming the attitude that problems are things to be fought against and conquered, try playing with the notion that an illness, or any other problem, may be a friend or a teacher at this particular time in your life. "Listen" to what this challenge has to teach you, or what it forces you to practice—like patience, courage, or creativity. Don't consider problems as something "bad" or "good"—just as "different" or "interesting."

Admittedly this attitude isn't easy to hold when times are really difficult. It takes gentle persistence to turn problems around and to make this approach to handling upsets a way of life. Why not begin now?

An Exercise for Beginners

Look out the window or step outside for a moment or two. Look at something, anything, in the natural environment—the sky, a cloud, a tree, a patch of earth. Soften your gaze, letting your eyes see each thing as if you have never seen it before. Be a beginner. Be an explorer. Let your curiosity about that thing grow. Now imagine that this is the very first and the very last time you will ever experience this gift. Absorb the impressions as fully as possible with all your senses and let yourself feel gratitude.

The Hebrew word *dayenu,* meaning "it is enough," captures the essence of living in gratitude for life. To live *dayenu* as a way of life is to be ready to embrace the mystery of the moment, fully, and then let it go. In this moment, all is a gift. One breath is precious, one smile, one day of seeing the sun. If there is no next moment, this attitude allows one to die freely, happily, with deep appreciation for all that has been and is.

The misery here is quite terrible; and yet, late at night . . . I often walk with a spring in my step along the barbed wire. And then time and again, it soars straight from my heart—I can't help it, that's just the way it is, like some elementary force the feeling that life is glorious and magnificent, and that one day we shall be building a whole new world.

Etty Hillesum, 1942,
Dutch Jew, died at Auschwitz

2 Inhabit Your Body and Love It

Twenty-four hours a day your body is talking to you—giving you feedback about what it needs for its survival, its pleasure, its growth, and its balance. Many of those messages go unnoticed or unheeded because of ignorance or lack of appreciation, or simply due to preoccupation with other matters. To inhabit your body means to start listening to what it is saying to you and to trust what you hear.

Few people escaped it as infants and toddlers—those wrinkled noses and parents' comments about the "mess" as diapers were changed. Perhaps you were admonished, "Don't touch yourself," and wondered at the concern this brought from your mom or dad. Undoubtedly it was drummed into you to keep yourself clean: "Scrub those hands; wash that hair; brush those teeth." Obviously the body was a fairly "dirty" thing! It wasn't to be trusted either. You were supposed to go to bed even when you didn't feel tired, to eat even when you weren't hungry, to wear a coat even when you weren't cold. If you weren't especially discouraged about your body's functions and the correctness of its feedback, you probably weren't exactly encouraged either.

It's not surprising that most people develop some dissociation from, and fear of, their own precious bodies and their natural processes. Typically, that dissociation endures throughout life. Even though the cultural norm encompasses an obsession with the body's appearance, few people know much about the body's workings. When was the concept of innate bodily knowledge or wisdom ever taught?

This shame and ignorance and dissociation, once learned, shows up as:

* being overweight
* being underweight
* an obsession with the body's shape
* a seeming lack of concern with the body's shape
* obsessions with cleanliness or tidiness
* fear of sexuality and intimacy
* physical symptoms like allergies, colds, or headaches
* emotional deadness

To inhabit your body means to be aware of it; to listen to and learn from its constant feedback; to accept and feel all things—whether pain or pleasure, happiness or grief; and to speak about yourself as if you were a whole being, especially when some "part" of you is in pain.

Our body will take care of us if given the slightest chance. It already has the best of nature within it and will survive if only we will let it, if we give it half the chance it has given and continues to give us each day.

RONALD J. GLASSER,
The Body is the Hero

Disease or pain is not the problem. More likely disease or pain is the body's attempt to solve the problem, a feedback of sorts that says something isn't working properly. And that "something" is probably much more than a rash or an ache. These symptoms may point to the need for a change in lifestyle, for emotional expression, or for spiritual guidance. The only way to find out what your body needs is to inhabit it.

You may feel as if you live outside and a little bit behind, or a few inches in front of, yourself, but not squarely aligned. Rushing ahead, or lagging behind, or listening to others instead of yourself, or saying yes when you mean no—in these and thousands of other ways you resign from yourself. Wellness is about "coming home"—taking up residence inside your own body once again.

If you want to know the secret of good health, set up home in your own body, and start loving yourself when there.

What Inhabiting Your Body Does for You

Inhabiting your body tunes you in to the twenty-four-hour-a-day feedback system through which your body offers valuable information on what it needs. You learn to listen to the body's reactions to different foods, different environments, different people. You discover your weak and vulnerable areas. These are the places where disease first shows up. For some people it is the throat. Others can literally feel the approach of a cold in their back and shoulders. Developing this kind of sensitivity to your built-in early warning system can often help you intervene (with extra rest and liquids, for example) and prevent an illness from taking hold.

When you inhabit your body, you can't help but develop a greater sense of awe and gratitude about it. The abilities and adaptabilities of the human organism are incredible! Unfortunately most people don't appreciate their body until something goes wrong with it. With heightened awareness, however, you may be inspired to study your body's processes more thoroughly in order to better interpret its signs. You may want to take better care of yourself and practice commonsense safety measures. You may learn to accept yourself as you are—strong, weak, healthy, in need, out of balance at times—a glorious series of contradictions. Your body is your home. Honoring your body builds self-esteem. You are remarkable!

Grace of movement is another advantage of inhabiting your body. You develop a more acute sense of where you begin, where you end, and how far you stretch in any direction. You understand the relationships between head and feet and legs and arms as you walk and move around. You don't move unconsciously as often, or walk ahead of yourself, so to speak. Rather you move from the inside out, conscious of what you are doing.

This sense of attunement to your body encourages you to live in the present moment, to feel whatever is going on within you, both physically and emotionally, whether pleasant or painful. You taste your food and experience your tears more fully. When you are stimulated by your natural environment, you require less stimulation from unhealthy sources. You don't need drugs or alcohol for excitement or excessive amounts of food to fill you up.

Meet Your Body

Take a moment to meet your feet again. Go ahead, kick off your shoes and lift one foot onto your lap and massage it, vigorously. Bring some energy into your foot. Now work on the other one. Remember that your feet have carried you, supported you for how many years of your life? They deserve some attention, some thanks. Try this: Stand up while you pay attention to your feet, without looking at them. Become aware of how your feet still work when you stand motionless, how they move as you walk, what they do as you sit down again. Come home to your feet!

Practice increased awareness of your whole body, as you've done for your feet. To start, place your hands gently on one area of your body. Bring your consciousness there. Sensitize yourself to what this area feels like under your hands, whether it is tight or relaxed, warm or cool; become aware of any fears or judgments or opinions you may have about this area of your body. Continue doing this for all of your body—internal organs as well as external parts.

Take off all your clothes and stand in front of a full-length mirror. Look at yourself. Keep looking. Look at everything. Observe what thoughts and judgments arise about yourself, then let go of all those opinions. See yourself as you are, without pretense, without masks, without defense. Keep looking; look long into your own eyes, but don't stay there the whole time. Bring compassion to this person. Keep looking, especially if you are tempted to turn away in boredom or disgust. Allow yourself plenty of time to do this, otherwise you may stop before receiving the full benefit of this exercise. Write down what you learned about yourself as you looked in the mirror.

Watch your language for ways in which you betray a sense of dissociation from, or hatred of, your body. Change your words from judgmental or condemnatory ones—"There goes that damn back, again"—to simple statements of fact—"My back hurts." If these feelings of self-deprecation are consistent and strong, get help from a counselor or therapist.

Body awareness and appreciation are integral to simple wellness. Refer back to this section as you continue working with the topics that follow.

The breath is life. That is why the yogi says that you "half-live" because you "half-breathe."

3 Breathe for Life

Adult humans normally breathe at the rate of one breath every six to eight seconds and inhale an average of sixteen thousand quarts of air each day. If nothing is done to restrict breathing, it will happen naturally and fully. But people continually inhibit natural breathing in many ways—poor posture, tight or binding clothes, "speed eating," exposure to noxious substances, smoking, lack of exercise, plus habitual patterns of emotional stress.

When breathing is obstructed or suppressed, the cells in the body do not receive the full amount of oxygen necessary to carry out their assigned functions. You may feel sleepy or irritable, or develop a headache. One reason that exercise is so valuable is that it forces you to breathe more fully, literally replenishing your dwindling supply of oxygen.

Hindus call it *prana*—the life force carried in the breath. Many languages use the same word for both breath and spirit, or life force.

In Hebrew, the word for soul or spirit is *rauch*. In Greek, it is *pneuma*. In Latin, *spiritus*. Each of these words also means "breath." In English, to inhale is to "inspire"—to take in the spirit. To exhale, or expire, means to release the spirit. All of life can be observed as a taking in and a giving out, of movement and rest, of controlling and letting go. The way you breathe is an excellent metaphor for the way you live your life.

The information and exercises recommended here encourage you to start paying attention to your breathing as a form of relaxation, stress reduction, and healing.

For additional help with stress reduction, see Chapter 9: Stretch Yourself (page 70), Chapter 11: Find Your Center—Learn to Meditate (page 83), Chapter 13: Welcome Necessary, Healing Touch—The Gift of Massage (page 92), Chapter 14: Lighten Up with Humor, Play, and Pleasure (page 100), Chapter 15: Move for the Health of It—Do Something Aerobic (page 109), and Chapter 26: Move Your Body and Move Your Soul (page 179).

Breath and Stress

Stress is inevitable—you need it to stand upright against the force of gravity. That's known as eustress, or positive stress, the kind that motivates you to get a job done on time or to do something that you thought was impossible.

When endangered by something in the environment or upset by disturbing thoughts—such as frightening expectations or memories like those associated with grief or panic—the body reacts to protect itself. It triggers a set of automatic responses, including increases in heart rate, in blood flow to the muscles, and in the rate of breathing. These responses are designed to energize the body to do battle, to run away, or to freeze. When the danger is real, the alarm state is necessary and important.

But there are many less dangerous forms of stress in your life that have the potential of wearing you down and causing a variety of health problems. Many people live in a constant state of alarm. "Stress plays some role in the development of every disease," writes Hans Selye, MD, in his classic work, *Stress without Distress.*

If stress is balanced with relaxation or attitude-change methods, the continual surge of energy supplied by the response to stress can be modified or even channeled for creative purposes. If stress levels remain high, disease and breakdown will often result.

Take a moment to recall some of the stressful situations in your life. Are there difficult people, either adults or children? Interruptions when you're trying to work or rest? Is there too much work, too little time? Are they driving in traffic? Smog and noise? Worries about your own health, or the health of someone in your family?

You may not be aware of it, but every tense situation, or even memories of tense situations, will cause a change in your breathing. Generally, the more stressed you feel, the more shallow your breathing will become. People who are under the strain of a serious loss frequently report that their chest feels locked, like they can't take a full breath. Almost every approach to relaxation and stress management focuses on attention to breathing.

Breathe to Relax

Here's an exercise that only takes a few minutes to complete, and you can do it imperceptibly almost anywhere, at any time.

1. If you can safely close your eyes, do that first. Otherwise, just stop talking and attend to your breathing.

2. Inhale, and as you inhale, say to yourself: "I am . . ." Exhale, and as you exhale, say to yourself: ". . . relaxed."

3. Continue repeating, "I am . . ." with each inhalation; ". . . relaxed" with each exhalation. Let the breathing

gradually become a little deeper, a little slower, but don't force it in any way. Just let it happen. As your mind begins to wander, gently bring it back to an awareness of breath and your statement, "I am . . . relaxed." Be easy on yourself. Continue doing this for a minute or two, longer if possible. Notice the overall effects of relaxation throughout your body.

More about Breath

While it is not possible or necessary to fully expand your lungs with every breath, you can heighten awareness of the breathing process, by intentionally creating a complete breath. Taking a full breath periodically uses the lungs to capacity and extracts great amounts of "life force" from the air.

Experience a Full Breath

Try this next exercise sitting, standing, and lying down. With gentle practice you will find that it becomes a smooth flow. Do it no more than about ten times consecutively unless you find the feeling of lightheadedness pleasurable.

1. Exhale deeply, contracting the belly.

2. Inhale slowly, expanding the belly first, then the chest, and finally raising the shoulders, slightly, up toward your ears. Hold this breath for a few comfortable seconds.

3. Exhale in the reverse pattern, slowly. Release your shoulders, relax your chest, relax your belly.

Breathing for Healing

Parents often sense that their child needs to breathe more fully to relieve panic or pain. The same is true for adults. Conscious breathing practices are now routinely taught in childbirth preparation classes. Anxiety intensifies pain, and the normal reaction is to tighten up when breathing. Breathing consciously not only will relieve tension and help quiet any fear, it can also relieve pain. So before you reach for the aspirins, the antacid tablets, or the telephone to call your doctor, do some breathing.

Here is a simple healing exercise:

1. Scan your body mentally, noticing how different areas are feeling.

Adult human beings breathe an average of 16,000 quarts of air each day.

2. As you inhale, imagine that you are breathing increased life into areas that feel tired, painful, tight, or "starved" in some way.

3. As you exhale, imagine that the tiredness, pain, and tightness are leaving with the expelled air.

4. Repeat for two or three minutes. Enjoy.

4 Befriend Your Feelings

Painful or confusing emotions are par for the course during a time of change, even when it's a positive, life-affirming change in the direction of overall health and wellbeing. If you are using this book to deal with a present illness or medical condition, you are especially likely to encounter strong or disturbing emotions. Anger, fear, unexpected tears, feelings of abandonment, and insecurity all may arise in a period of questioning or transition. If you have had surgery or are taking medication, emotional fluctuations are even more common.

Since there is no way to separate body from mind from emotions, any small changes you are making to orient yourself toward high-level wellness have the potential of arousing feelings, and it is not always easy to plot the link between actions and the emotions they trigger. You may not see a connection between practicing a new breathing exercise, for instance, and a feeling of sadness that washes over you like a wave.

In order to move toward something new, you must often let go of something old. "Letting go" is one way to describe loss, and loss is always accompanied by grief, however slight. When you stop smoking, you may feel the loss of that special rendezvous you had every morning with your fellow smokers. If you change your diet, you may feel resentment at watching others indulge freely in foods that you now avoid. Feelings are part and parcel of a life undergoing change. Be assured. You are not going crazy. You are right on schedule.

What's the Problem with Feelings?

In many cultures there is a great deal of confusion about feelings—especially the strong or painful ones. TV and movies portray people expressing themselves passionately and violently, but in everyday life in the American culture there isn't much permission to rock the emotional boat. It is often considered a sign of weakness to display fear or grief overtly. The desired countenance is one of strength and control, and children are taught, at least by example, to be brave, to act "cool." People are very uncomfortable when those around them "break down." Others think there is something wrong with themselves when they feel depressed.

The cultural norms about anger are really confused. People overlook and sometimes even expect the exchange of angry words in public among strangers, and may applaud it as a motivator to sports and competition and war. The same people then express disbelief or horror when a close friend or family member expresses anger with them or learns that battering and other forms of abuse are going on close to home. Some people are shocked to discover how much anger they have, and try to repress it, while others use anger as a way to eliminate any emotional energy that they don't know how to handle.

Joy and exuberance are generally acceptable as long as they are "controlled." It's all right to sing in church or to dance at a party or nightclub. But you might be thought crazy if you burst into song in a department store or dance ecstatically in the town square. There are many unwritten rules about expressing feelings.

Stop for a moment and recall some of the messages you got about feelings when you were young.

What was held up to you as model behavior? Do any of these statements sound familiar? "Don't get too excited or silly; somebody's bound to get hurt." "Don't cry. That's for babies." "Don't ever say you hate anyone." "Keep going, no matter how bad you feel." "Just think happy thoughts and everything will be fine." "Don't expect anything, and you won't be disappointed." It is little wonder that many people have grown up to be emotionally confused and wounded adults.

There is a heavy price to be paid when feelings are denied or repressed. Lethargy, boredom, and a sense of deadness toward life may be the sorry consequence. When this happens, bigger and stronger forms of stimulation are required to feel happy and alive. Some people drink, others drive recklessly. Paradoxically, some people get seriously ill as a way to get attention and still feel alive.

An equally heavy price is exacted when feelings are overindulged and dramatized as a means of justifying ourselves or manipulating others. Some people punish themselves with their own anger or guilt; they close themselves off completely from help, and therefore from the healing potential of human relationships, withdrawing from others to obsess about their own wounds.

Those who are unaccustomed to dealing with feelings in healthy ways often seek out other means to cover their feelings, or to distract themselves from feeling at all. At the first inklings of pain, fear, or loneliness, they may turn to alcohol, food, drugs, TV, unhealthy relationships, or compulsive work. Thus, bigger problems, more pain, and more fear are created in a terrified attempt to avoid pain and fear.

Repressing emotions out of fear or pain may lead to a habit of trying to control and dominate others as well. This form of relating—the stern teachers who won't tolerate the enthusiasm of children; the rigid bosses who only want things done their way—has, in some domains, become the norm. These highly controlled individuals, however, are emotionally unwell. Inner strength and integrity come with the ability and willingness to acknowledge and/or express emotions freely, to use emotional energy constructively. The result is partnership, rather than a dominant or submissive role in relationship to others.

In considering the connection between wellness and feelings, we have seen what happens with clients and students when "emotional" energy—anger and sadness in particular—gets blocked. Depression is common with people who do not allow themselves to experience rage or grief. And depression will weaken the immune system, making the whole body more susceptible to disease. Other people literally create a body armor by severely tightening muscles in an attempt to defend against painful emotions. Such armored bodies are more apt to develop symptoms of chronic pain and crippling disease.

How to Deal with Feelings

Adopt the attitude that feelings are natural and normal. This is a primary healing attitude. Strong feelings are not indicators of something "bad." Feelings have no morality. They just are. Even if you are uncomfortable with them, accept strong emotions as valuable feedback telling you that something in your life is in need of attention. And the best attention is gentle acceptance. Befriend the emotional parts of yourself.

✻ WRITE ABOUT YOUR FEELINGS. Express and explore your feelings on paper. Write an angry letter and then tear it up, or compose a poem about your grief. There are many books that suggest ways to use writing for self-help; see the resources at the end of the book.

* DRAW OR PAINT OR DANCE YOUR FEELINGS. This is a healthy way to defuse potentially explosive emotions and to soothe painful ones. When you've expressed yourself creatively, you may have a whole new perspective on the situation and may be in a more balanced place from which to speak to others.

* EXERCISE VIGOROUSLY. Exert yourself. Exercising, even brisk walking, will take the emphasis off the worrying mind and encourage fuller breathing, which is a powerful healer of emotional wounds. Try digging a hole and voicing your emotional pain into that hole. Then when you are finished, fill the hole back up with soil.

See Chapter 6: Watch Your Words—Avoid Illness Programming (page 52) and Chapter 29: Put Yourself in the Picture of Health (page 193) to practice mental visualization.

* TALK ABOUT YOUR FEELINGS. If you are confused, you can always start a conversation with a friend by saying, "I am not sure what I'm feeling," and proceed from there. Your listeners may not have answers for you, but the process of speaking opens the door for both clarification and support.

* CHANGE YOUR MIND. Because thoughts arouse feelings, if you change what you are focusing on or thinking about, your feelings will change accordingly. When you are feeling frightened or inadequate, remember a time when you were strong and competent and create a

mental image to support that. This type of imagery is used in many healing disciplines.

* SURRENDER YOUR FEELINGS. Give them over, along with the rest of your life, to a higher power.

Recognize and Accept Your Emotions

Here is a simple exercise that will help you sensitize yourself to how and where emotions affect your body, and will encourage you to accept emotions as natural expressions of your being. You can do this exercise alone or invite a friend to help you.

1. Sit or lie down in a comfortable place. Close your eyes and breathe slowly and deeply to help you relax.

2. Repeat the following phrases five times each, very slowly but energetically, so you can really generate the mood of the phrase. (Or ask your friend to say them for you.) As you speak, focus all of your attention on the physical sensations that these words evoke.

* I am scared.
* I give up.
* I hate you.
* I love you.

* Please don't leave me.
* No, no, no.
* Yes, yes, yes.

Add an emotionally charged phrase of your own. Try to sense where these various emotions "live" in your body and how they affect you physically.

3. Repeat the exercise, but this time let the feelings come and go as if they were currents of air blowing through you. You can learn to feel your feelings without identifying with them so closely that they overpower you. Let fear be there. Let discouragement be there. Don't try to chase them away. Look at them. Then move on to the next emotional statement.

4. Share with your friend, or write about, what you have learned as a result of doing this.

5 Discover What You Already Know

Wellness starts with the recognition that your body is wise, your mind is wise, and your soul is wise. You may not always honor that wisdom in yourself, but it is there nonetheless. You are at the leading edge of over five billion years of evolution. You are a being of amazing resources. It's time to discover that.

Humans have an insatiable hunger for answers and cures, and show great persistence in their searches, which may take them around the world and back. Yet in looking "out there," they overlook, dismiss, and even demean the obvious—the knowledge that lies within.

Experts and guides are valuable in all aspects of life. But the trouble comes when too much responsibility is shifted onto these experts, these doctors and teachers, and intuition and self-understanding are ignored. Giving away personal power to an ever-growing army of "professionals" puts us on the well-worn path to a power-robbed existence. Such reliance easily becomes a source of confusion when the advice of one specialist seems to contradict that of another.

One simple way to practice self-responsibility is to acknowledge what you already know about your own life and health. You have a basic sense of what's good for you and what isn't. By looking within and asking yourself some simple questions, you can access information for your own wellbeing. If you are currently seeing doctors or other helping professionals, share this additional, valuable information with them. It will help

The next major advances in health of the American people will come from the assumption of individual responsibility for one's own health and a necessary change in lifestyle for the majority of Americans.

John H. Knowles,
former president, Rockefeller Foundation

to move you out of the role of passive patient and into a partnership with a healing team.

In a classic study conducted by psychologists Ellen Langer of Harvard and Judith Rodin of Yale, elderly residents in a nursing home were given plants to care for and were encouraged to do more for themselves instead of letting the staff take over all their responsibilities. Another group of patients, of similar age and disability, received no such encouragement for self-responsibility. Within three weeks, there was significant improvement in the health and vitality levels of the first group. Eighteen months later, even more dramatic findings were revealed. The death rate in the "increased responsibility" group was half that of the other group.

This is only one example from a growing body of scientific research that supports the theory that individuals who have choices in managing and directing their own lives stay healthier, live longer, and heal faster than those who do not.

An Experience in Discovering

1. Have pencil and paper handy. Now, begin by letting yourself relax. Sit back and take a few slow breaths. Close your eyes, if you wish, to help achieve an inward

focus, and just rest for a minute or so. When you feel at ease, open your eyes. Working quickly now, make a list of things that encourage your health and wellness. You can write out each response in a complete sentence, or simply use a word, phrase, or symbol to capture your idea. For instance:

* I know that more outdoor exercise helps me to work better.
* I know . . .
* I know . . .

2. Next, make another list, this time focusing on things that discourage health and wellness for you. For instance:

* I know that eating in the car as I'm driving is not conducive to my digestion.
* I know that . . .
* I know that . . .

3. Expand this self-discovery by writing yourself a letter about your current state of illness or health. Write as one best friend to another. Address any other issues that may be particularly troublesome for you at this time and don't hesitate to write about the changes you

want and what you know will support you in making those changes. For example:

> *Dear Janet,*
> *I know you've had a lot of pain recently, and I want to encourage you to keep up your exercise program, which really seems to help. There are some other things that might be beneficial for you, like . . .*
>
> *Love, Janet*

You will gain maximum benefit from the exercises suggested above by repeating them periodically. For instance, try writing a letter to yourself every day for a week or more. Remember, as you write, that your health or illness is influenced by your state of mind, your emotions, and your spirit. Consider all aspects of yourself as you write your letters. You may find it helpful to write about your fears, your grief, your imagined weaknesses, and your negative opinions about yourself. Write also about your insights and intuitions, your dreams and plans, your day-to-day learning about questions of being and meaning.

Doing this kind of honest self-exploration will gradually reveal more of your own inner wisdom. This will give you the confidence to trust yourself as the expert on your own healing. You can begin to shape your life in new ways that promote greater health and wellness. You can speak self-reliantly to your doctor or other experts about what you know about yourself.

Take That First Step Today

Now that you are off to a good start by discovering what you already know, it is time to act on that knowledge. Please don't discourage yourself by attempting an instant overhaul of all of your life patterns. Habits have built up over years and will take time to change. What is one step that you can take today to encourage your wellness? Write it down. Do it. And give yourself a pat on the back for taking one small step toward health and wellbeing. For instance:

* I will walk outdoors, vigorously, for ten minutes today.
* I will refrain from eating sugary snacks or desserts today and have fresh fruit or nuts and raisins instead.
* I will . . .

6 Watch Your Words—
Avoid Illness Programming

The world is such-and-such or so-and-so only because we tell ourselves that that is the way it is.

CARLOS CASTANEDA

The childhood rhyme that says, "Sticks and stones may break my bones, but words can never hurt me," is far from true. Words can literally kill. In the introduction to Norman Cousins's *The Healing Heart,* Dr. Bernard Lown, professor of cardiology at Harvard, tells a story that illustrates the power of words. A woman he was treating displayed severe panic-type reactions upon hearing the physician say that she had TS (tricuspid stenosis, a condition of obstructed blood flow in the heart). The woman interpreted this as "terminal situation" and reacted accordingly. She developed massive lung congestion and died from heart failure the same day.

Of course, this is an extreme case. Nevertheless, it is true that your words create your world. As you look around your surroundings, you are talking to yourself about everything you see. Your language structures your reality. Furniture and pictures are not good or bad in and of themselves. They become beautiful or ugly, valuable or worthless, based on your descriptions of them. The clothes you're wearing are fashionable or dowdy, depending on your judgment of them. So too with your health. If you tell yourself that starving a fever will help relieve it, it probably will. If you say that arthritis and senility are inevitable, they probably will be. People tend to find what they have told themselves to expect.

Where Our Illness Programming Originates

Your brain operates like a highly sophisticated computer, storing every experience you have ever had in your subconscious. Brain research reveals that subjects can describe minute details of events that happened to them as children; clinical hypnosis allows people to remember things that the conscious mind may have filed away long ago. The body acts and reacts on the basis of its previous programming, even without the mind's conscious acknowledgement. So many of your illness reactions and fears of today are the results of messages you received as a child. You keep these old programs in place with unconscious self-talk and reinforce them with new input from contemporary sources.

✻ CHILDHOOD ROLE MODELS. You may have watched Mom or Dad start every day with a dose of aspirin for pain or end every day with a few drinks to handle stress. You wondered why certain topics, like sex and death, made adults very uncomfortable and why certain words, like *cancer,* were never used.

* DIRECT COMMANDS FROM PARENTS AND OTHERS. "You'll fall." "Oh, you'll get sick." "You'll cut yourself." And sure enough, you probably did!

* REWARDS FOR ILLNESS OR FOR BEING IN PAIN. You may have received special attention like physical nurturing, been allowed to stay home from school, or been given candy and ice cream or gifts.

* TV, MAGAZINES AND NEWSPAPERS, AND BILLBOARDS. The media constantly supplies direct illness messages such as "The winter cold season is here!" or "Don't worry about overeating, as long as you have those little white mints to fight indigestion." Even more insidious are the implied messages, like "Cancer is inevitable and will always mean death."

* DAILY CONVERSATIONS. Some people constantly complain about their own symptoms and the ill health of those around them.

* SELF-DESIGNED, SELF-DESTRUCTIVE MENTAL PICTURES of your pain or disease. Humans are image-making creatures. Constantly and, for the most part, unconsciously, your imagination creates internal images of things that it cannot see, hear, feel, taste, or touch.

Hearing the word *ulcer,* you will form a mental picture (or some other internal sensory image—not everyone creates a visual image) of an ulcer, even if you have never seen one. It may not be an accurate representation, but if the idea of an ulcer is a troubling thought for you, your stomach may tighten up nonetheless.

Self-Programming That Heals

If negative messages and images can worsen a condition, doesn't it make sense that life-affirming messages will help to heal it? This is not just some fantasy. Research in the field of psychoneuroimmunology verifies what folk healers have known for centuries—that thoughts and emotions directly affect the strength of the immune system. The immune system is the first line of defense against disease. If you can strengthen your immune system consciously, through imagery and nurturing self-talk, you have a much better chance of maintaining the health of your whole body.

Man is troubled not by events themselves but by the views he takes of them.

EPICTETUS, *c. 100 C.E.*

Imagery and nurturing self-talk are used with great success to control pain. In a study conducted at the University of California, Irvine, many patients suffering from chronic back pain received long-term relief by using a variety of self-control techniques, including consciously slowing down their breathing, creating positive mental imagery, and repeating nurturing self-talk, which reinforced pain-free feelings. Similar approaches are routinely used at pain centers as well as in natural childbirth, surgical preparation, mental rehearsal for sports performances, and even for the treatment of burns.

Motivational programs and stress management courses universally include some sort of training in the use of nurturing self-talk or affirmations. These encouraging sentences are repeated many times in the course of a day, and more often during times of discouragement or stress to counteract the effects of negative thinking, to inspire relaxation, and to build confidence.

You no longer have to be at the mercy of your own illness programming. By becoming aware of it, you will learn whether it is helping you or hindering you. You can then make some conscious choices. It is within your control to design new, healing images and to choose words that will support a healthier inner and outer environment.

Exercises in Reprogramming

Start listening for your illness programming. Learn how you talk to yourself about whatever you're doing or not doing. (For example, after sitting at your computer for an hour or so, your lower back may hurt. You might say something to yourself like "Oh, no. I still have that bad back. What a pain. If it's this bad now, it will be a lot worse when I'm older." These negative tape loops discourage, depress, and almost always disempower you by reinforcing the belief that the pain was inevitable.) Listen also for internal messages of self-deprecation that tell you what you are doing is not good enough, such as "You'll never win. You're all wrong. There you go again." For a day or two, write down these messages whenever you notice them. Awareness is the first step toward change.

Create a simple, nurturing affirmation that declares health and wholeness. For instance: "I am growing in strength and self-mastery easily and peacefully." Repeat it morning, noon, and night, and whenever you notice negative self-talk. Design your affirmation to address the issue you most want to change. For example, if you are working on eating more fresh fruits and vegetables, your affirmation might state: "I am enjoying the way my body feels when eating fresh foods. I appreciate myself for the care I show in eating more nutritious foods."

Draw a picture of yourself being healthy and whole. Make several copies of this picture and put it around your house.

Life's door, love's door, God's door—they all open when you are playful. They all become closed when you become serious.

Osho

Put cues in your environment, like colored stickers or dots. Place them where you will see them often. Each time you spot a cue, remind yourself of your new programs and new pictures.

Unplug your TV and stop reading the news for at least a month. Notice any effect on your overall health.

Read between the lines whenever you read, watch TV, or have a conversation, to discover the hidden illness programs around you. Write them down.

In wilderness is the preservation of the world.

HENRY DAVID THOREAU

7 Connect with Nature

The human body needs the touch of nature along with the touch of human skin. Yet too many people have dulled their senses and thus silenced that need. It's easy to go several months without ever touching the earth, as most of our activities involve walking on pavement as we move from home to car to office to grocery store and back again. When was the last time you sat down on the ground or touched the earth in some way?

Physical contact with soil, natural waters, sunlight, and fresh air is healing. When stress has built up to the danger point, a trip to the ocean or mountains, or even a walk around the block, is often all you need to restore perspective. Beyond that, contact with nature keeps you apprised of your place in the ecological system. Many of nature's forces are stronger than an individual human, just as many species are more vulnerable than humankind. This humbling perspective keeps the big picture in mind.

Start Today

Here are some simple ways to connect with nature again:

* Go barefoot. Feel the grass or the gravel or the hard-packed earth under your feet. Wade in a rain puddle, or walk barefoot in the snow for a new sensation!
* Grow plants or flowers and let your fingers touch the earth.
* Keep living green plants and flowers around your house.
* Get outdoors, if only for a few moments a day. Let the sunlight touch you and warm you. (For longer periods in the sun, be sure to wear protective clothing and hats.) In the heart of a city, it is still possible to find green zones.

* Listen to the sounds of nature—the wind blowing, rain falling, birds chirping—even in the midst of an urban environment.
* Prepare your meals using fresh and raw foods whenever possible, or bake your own bread. Carefully handling the fruits of the field reminds you of your connection to the earth.
* Practice the Native American way of adapting yourself to nature, rather than trying to make nature adapt to you. For example, avoid dependency on air-conditioning in hot weather. In cold weather, keep the heat in your home at 68°F (20°C) or lower.
* When you are around young children, use language that communicates a healthy respect for the power of nature and a sense of awe at its beauty and mystery. Avoid teaching them that soil is dirty or that any creatures (even so-called vermin) are bad.
* Exercise outdoors as much as possible. Take a hike. Go for a bike ride instead of driving your car to the corner store. Rollerblade in the park, or get a group of friends together for a ball game or a kite-flying party.
* Plan your vacations for maximum enjoyment of the outdoors (with minimal environmental impact).

See Chapter 23: Befriend the Earth (page 161) to learn more about adapting yourself to nature.

Even a one-day family trip with a picnic can be a tremendously healthy break in your normal routine.

8 Set Goals for the Changes You Want to Make

If your approach to life is mainly one of "going with the flow," you're likely to find yourself being washed down the stream, backward.

To have any real sense of getting somewhere, it's helpful to know where you're starting from and where you want to go. Goal setting is a dynamic tool for getting things done, and helps you clarify what is important in your life, what your priorities are. And it aids self-esteem. By setting goals you are resisting the mentality that says you are a victim in life. Instead, you affirm your choice for self-responsibility: "I am responsible for my life and health" and "I am a worthwhile person."

Goals are like maps—they keep you on course. More than that, goals are like magnets—they tend to attract things that help get them accomplished. It's almost magical at times, the way this works. When you put down in words what you want to achieve, you immediately start to see or remember the resources that are all around you.

Many people make lists of the things they have to do that day or that week. When they cross some items off, they have a feeling of accomplishment. Even if they only get through half the list, they still feel good knowing that they've moved forward.

There is power in setting goals, so tap into that power now.

Small Changes—An Exercise in Setting Goals

People often overwhelm themselves by tackling a goal that they think they "should" achieve. They set their sights too high and then quit completely when they don't make the grade. It helps to make a distinction between the goals you think you want and the goals to which you *will really commit.*

1. Read back over the letters and lists you generated in Chapter 5: Discover What You Already Know (page 46). Star any items that you really want to change or work on in some way. Add any new ones that occur to you. Call this selection of starred items and additions your "Want List."

If you didn't do the exercises offered in that section, draw up a Want List now, noting aspects of your life that you know are affecting your overall health. For example: the people, behaviors, circumstances, and environments that encourage or discourage your wellness.

2. Now look over your Want List and put a double star next to any items that you are ready to change or work on in some way right now. Write down those items in complete sentences that express your willingness to act. For example:

I am ready and willing to commit to making a change in my habit of driving over the speed limit.

I am ready and willing to. . . .

3. Prioritize your commitment statements.

4. Starting with your top priority item, brainstorm for a moment or two about any preliminary steps you will need to take before you can start working directly on your goal. For example, will you need to purchase some special equipment, shop at a different food store, start reading a book on nutrition, get some instruction in

weight-bearing exercise, or have a consultation with your doctor? Write these steps down.

Now set up a schedule for accomplishing these preliminaries. Assigning specific dates, times, places, or methods to these items will maximize the likelihood of your follow-through.

5. Next, make a Resource List of the people, places, and things that are available to help you in fulfilling your commitment. For example:

My children, I can ask them to remind me of my commitment when they see I am breaking it.

6. Determine the length of time that you will work on this goal. An hour? A day? Two weeks? And decide how often you will check your progress and when you will reevaluate your goal. For example:

For the next three days I will get up a half-hour earlier each morning and take a vigorous twenty-minute walk before having breakfast. I will evaluate my progress (how I felt during the walk; how that exercise affected my overall energy throughout the day) on the evening of the third day and decide then whether I will continue the walks.

7. Keep encouraged by always congratulating yourself for any advances you've made, no matter how small. Remember, the bigger your goals, the bigger the challenge and the greater the likelihood that you will have setbacks. That's a normal part of growing and changing. Maintain a nonjudgmental attitude toward yourself for what you have not yet accomplished and honor yourself for what you have done.

8. Work on only one or, at most, two goals at a time. When you have established them as natural parts of your lifestyle, then move on to other goals.

For anything to make a difference in a person's life, an insight must be followed up by action.

JIM ZARVOS

Setting Goals for Life

At the same time that you are building your self-mastery by working on short-term goals, it is very helpful to map out a bigger picture for yourself—a plan for your life and health for years into the future. The following exercise will guide you in this process.

1. Take four blank sheets of paper. Head them as follows: 1) Where/how I want my life and health to be five years from today; 2) Where/how I want my life and health to be two years from today; 3) Where/how I want my life

and health to be six months from today; and 4) How I would spend the next six months if I knew for sure they would be my last.

As you work on these lists, be creative. Ask yourself: "What would I have/do/be if I had no limitation (like time, money, or job responsibilities)?" Work on each sheet as quickly as possible, taking no more than fifteen minutes for each.

2. Read over all you have written and look for goals that are repeated or strongly expressed. These will be your priorities.

3. Put the exercise aside for a few days and then repeat Step 1. Compare the results, looking for the goals that were clearly priorities in both writings. This exercise helps you ascertain your values and plan the next steps in your life journey.

4. Focus on one or more of your strongest goals and create a Road Map—a series of action steps that will bring your dream into form within the desired time frame. For example: If your goal is to have a significantly stronger body in two years, write down the preliminary

steps you will need to take to gather the necessary resources and information to start this. Taking a trip to the library to get a book on nutrition or making a phone call to a local gym might be a good beginning here.

If you already know how to go about getting what you want, simply list the action steps and a schedule. For example, write down what type of exercise program you will use and when you will start it; what modification you will make to your diet and when and how you will do this; and so on.

Approach those "impossible" goals by breaking them down into workable daily actions. Or, think of it this way: How do you create a garden where there wasn't one before? You start today by removing one rock at a time.

5. Plan for frequent reviews and reevaluations to ensure that your steps are realistic and to keep yourself encouraged along the way.

6. Share your goals with friends and invite their support in helping you stay on task, or join a support group that has similar goals. Creating a support network is invaluable to your journey. In fact, it may be essential.

Traps to Avoid

Hundreds of different mental messages, including doubts and fears, will arise to discourage you from designing any goals and from sticking with them when you hit your first temporary setback. Some of these messages might include:

* "I already tried this once, and it didn't work."
* "People are always trying to get me to set goals. I'll show them who's boss!"
* "What if I set a goal and then don't make it? I'll feel worse."
* "What if I do make it? Will people expect me to do it all the time?"
* "It's a waste of time to make plans. Nobody can predict the future. Just take whatever comes."

These messages are dangerous because each of them is partially true. Of course you can't predict the future. And people probably will expect more of you if they see you are a person who can achieve a goal. These messages can become self-defeating if you give them energy, but remember that they are only thoughts. Don't let them stop you. Keep moving ahead. The difference between a life of greatness and a life of mediocrity is that great people move beyond their limitations, while the mediocre sit around talking about them.

Part II
loosening up

*

Too often you are challenged without being adequately prepared. It's like running or climbing a mountain without warming up first. Part II will help you loosen up. You will be guided in ways to nurture yourself in preparation for the challenges that lie ahead.

In Part II you will learn how to:

* make physical stretching a part of your everyday routine
* eliminate much of the unnecessary tension you carry around
* center yourself through meditation
* use water for healing and nourishment
* give yourself a healing massage
* take a break from seriousness and laugh more

9 Stretch Yourself

Stretching is the important link between the sedentary life and the active life. It keeps the muscles supple, prepares you for movement, and helps you make the daily transition from inactivity to vigorous activity without undue strain.

Bob Anderson, MD, *Stretching*

One of the simplest and most effective ways to release tension and energize yourself is to take time out for a good stretch. You can stretch in almost any position, and, in fact, a good stretch before you get out of bed in the morning is a fine way to start the day. Developing the habit of stretching frequently throughout the day will make a big difference in how you feel.

Stretch yourself, right now.

Good.

Now take a deep, full breath, and stretch again in a different way than you did the first time.

Terrific.

Most people claim that stretching feels good. It helps release muscle tension almost immediately, which results in an overall sense of relaxation. As it breaks up energy blockages in the body, stretching allows for better circulation. It improves your range of motion, too. As you ease into a stretch, you literally reach farther. Stretching is also a way to increase self-awareness. Focusing on how different body parts feel when they are being stretched increases your power of concentration and heightens your awareness of internal feedback. With growing self-awareness comes a greater sense of self-control. The more you honor your body, the more you listen to what it wants and needs, the more you will appreciate it. And this just naturally blossoms into greater self-esteem.

When you stretch, don't make jerky, quick, or bouncing movements. Instead, ease into your stretches in a smooth, relaxed way and hold the stretched posture externally while you internally release the muscles. If you feel any pain, stop. Stretching that causes pain can lead to serious injury if muscle tissues lose elasticity and tear. "No pain, no gain" should be understood metaphorically, not literally, where stretching is concerned. Breathe consciously while stretching and imagine that you are actually breathing into the parts of the body being stretched.

Refer to Chapter 3: Breathe for Life (page 32) for instructions on breathing fully.

Start Your Day with a Stretch

Choose from among the movements suggested below or develop your own routine for starting your day with a stretch. Each of these stretches can be done in bed.

1. Lying on your back, with your legs flat on the bed and pointing your toes away from your head, stretch your legs as far as they will go toward the foot of the bed. If

you have enough space on your bed, stretch your arms straight back behind your head with fingers pointing away from your feet. Otherwise, stretch your arms out at a ninety-degree angle to your body. Extend your fingers and toes. Hold for ten seconds. Release, flexing your fingers and toes. Repeat two or three times.

2. Lying on your back, reach for the ceiling. Extend and then flex your fingers. Tense, relax, and shake your arms.

3. Bring your knees up toward your chest. Grasp them with your arms. In this position, roll to your left, then back to center, then roll to your right and back to center. Repeat as often as is fun. Release your knees. Extend your legs.

4. Still lying on your back, with your knees bent and your feet flat on the bed, alternately arch your lower back for five seconds then flatten your lower back to the bed again for five seconds. Repeat three or four times, or as feels good.

5. With your knees bent and your feet flat on the bed, slowly rotate your pelvis clockwise three times, as you

keep your knees pointing toward the ceiling. Make small movements. Rotate counterclockwise three times in the same manner.

6. Bend your knees, placing your feet flat on the bed. Raise your buttocks off the bed. Hold for a count of three. Lower your buttocks back onto bed. Repeat three or four times.

7. Inhale as you turn your head to the right slowly, lowering your right ear to the bed. Exhale as you return head to center. Repeat, turning your head to the left. Do this three or four times. Relax.

8. Roll over onto your stomach. Bend your knees and bring the heels of your feet up toward your buttocks. If you are able to, grasp your ankles or heels and pull your heels toward your buttocks. Hold for ten to twenty seconds. Lower your feet to the bed again. Repeat twice.

9. Still on your stomach, keeping your chest lowered, ease your upper body back until your thighs and knees are under your chest and your buttocks are resting on your lower legs. This kneeling-type pose is sometimes

called the Baby Pose in yoga. Reach back and hold your heels or your ankles if you can. Tuck your head down toward your chest. Feel your neck and back stretch with this one. Hold for ten to twenty seconds. Enjoy it. Release.

10. Let go of your feet. Raise your head and straighten your back, coming to a sitting posture by either sitting back on your legs and feet, or putting your legs over the side of the bed and placing your feet on the floor. Look in the direction of the sunrise. Smile and greet the day. Get out of bed.

The All-Day Stretching Habit

Feeling tense and depleted at the end of a day doesn't have to be the norm. You can use stretching exercises throughout the day, before and after every activity you perform, as a way of releasing stress and of getting back in touch with yourself.

* DRIVING YOUR CAR TODAY? Stretch before you get behind the wheel. Stretch as you drive. Take a deep breath and stretch your neck, your shoulders, your face. Adjust the position of your back frequently. On long-distance drives, stop every hour or so for a stretch break.

* OFFICE WORK? Try isometric contractions as you sit at your desk. Inhale, tighten the muscles in your arms, shrug your shoulders up, extend your elbows, and form a fist. Feel the tension mount from your fingers all the way up to your shoulders. Hold for a few seconds, then release completely. These exercises can be done with your shoulders, back, legs, or your whole body. And they can be done so subtly that nobody around you will know what you're doing (unless you want to invite them to feel better, too).

* USE EVERYDAY ACTIVITIES AS A WAY OF STRETCHING OUT. Instead of mindlessly reaching for that box on the top shelf, imagine that you are doing a stretching exercise. Take a breath. Move smoothly. Hold the maximum stretch for twenty to thirty seconds. When making your bed, do a series of stretches. You can be creative and have fun, literally making a dance out of everything you do.

Hatha Yoga

The ancient discipline of hatha yoga combines slow movements and stretching postures with breathing exercises. Yoga is never supposed to be a huffing-puffing ordeal, thus making it especially beneficial for the handicapped and the elderly, for anyone who has not exercised in a long time, or for those who suffer from chronic pain. The postures not only stretch the body, they also stimulate the nervous system and endocrine glands; activate circulation, digestion, and elimination; help to balance the energy flow in the right and left sides of the brain, and therefore in the rest of the body; align the vertebrae; and promote a deepened sense of inner peace.

There are yoga exercises for every part of the body, from the eyes to the toes. Try this simple stretch called the Lion Pose, which is designed to relax tension you hold in your face. It feels great and looks silly, so it should make you smile!

The Lion Pose

1. Inhale.

2. While you forcefully exhale, open your mouth as wide as you can, stick out your tongue, open your eyes as wide as they will go, and stretch your arms down with fingers stiff and spread apart.

3. Hold this posture, without breathing, for a few seconds. Notice how your facial muscles feel.

4. Release the posture. Close your mouth and inhale deeply. Your abdomen should expand as you do so.

5. Exhale slowly through your nose.

6. Repeat two more times.

Does your face feel warmer or more energized? Are you more aware of facial muscles that you never knew you had? Did you feel a stretch in other parts of your body as you did that pose with your face?

If you are interested in learning more about hatha yoga, refer to the books on yoga listed in the resources at the end of the book or contact your public library. Yoga classes are often taught at fitness centers.

10 Loosen Up Your Belt and Everything Else

Imagine trying to blow up a balloon that is knotted in the middle, and you'll have some idea of the stress created in your body when tight clothing restricts normal breathing. A tight and contracted abdomen, moreover, will adversely affect normal posture, digestion, and elimination.

Unfortunately, fashion trends generally are not motivated by a human being's organic needs. Figure-controlling pantyhose and tight jeans are big business and not easily dismissed, yet they take their toll by fostering poor breathing habits. This can lead to a whole range of imbalanced conditions from hemorrhoids to circulation problems to headaches and more.

How can the diaphragm possibly do its job of expanding if the abdominal muscles refuse to move? Your body will compensate by breathing from the upper chest, but the result is only a half breath. And tightness in the lower body will be worsened by the lack of oxygen flow to that area. No wonder you may feel sleepy or in pain after only a brief period of sitting at your desk.

Take a moment to mentally scan your whole body from head to toe. Be aware of your clothing. Feel tightness anywhere? Bra? Belt? Shirt collar? Tie or scarf? Shoes? Now take a deep breath and feel any additional areas of tightness or restriction caused by your clothing. Is your body temperature comfortable? Are you too hot? Too cool? Loosen your belt or any tight or binding clothing, or take off a layer, and take another deep breath. What are you aware of now?

Next consider your posture. Is it possible to breathe fully without strain in the position you are currently in? Where does the breath get stuck; what parts of the body feel tight inside as you try to breathe deeply? Can you adjust your posture to accommodate a fuller, more relaxed breath? Do so if you wish.

Beyond Breathing

There is more to this issue than restrictive clothes and poor breathing habits. What about high heels, which are known to cause misalignment in the body? What about the position and design of office furniture, the height of keyboards or computer screens? These things can usually be adjusted to accommodate better posture or to give the body more room to move. Often people put up with unnecessary pain because they don't stop to think about how easily they could change their situation.

Let's not overlook the issue of clothing fabrics and how these restrict the skin's ability to breathe. Many skin disorders and rashes are simply the results of irritation and poor ventilation caused by clothing. Popular synthetics, such as dacron and polyester, are made of smooth fibers that can be woven very tightly. These fabrics may resist wrinkling, but they don't breathe. Since the body invisibly eliminates a substantial portion of waste products through the skin, open-weave fabrics like cotton and wool are more healthful.

Many people wear a particular uniform or clothing style at their jobs. You can still dress in healthier and looser clothing with careful shopping and a little creativity. Many shoe companies now carry styles that are sensibly designed yet suitable for business wear, and comfortable, neatly tailored clothing is available in natural fabrics.

Get in the habit of tuning in to your body, becoming aware of tightness or pain that builds up or surprises you as you go through your day. This tension can take many forms. Some people walk around with their shoulders up around their ears; others keep their buttock muscles constantly contracted. You may wrinkle your forehead and give yourself wrinkles and headaches; you may grit your teeth and actually grind them down or create a chronic tension in your jaw; you may clench your fists, often to compensate for an unwillingness to express emotion in more direct ways.

Besides trapping the tension in your body, all of these unconscious gestures expend energy. Become aware of how tightly you hold your toothbrush, or your pencil, or the steering wheel of your car. Over time, these unconscious habits can take their toll. They can hurt your body, as can happen with overly vigorous toothbrushing, which can wear away tooth enamel. Sitting tensely behind the wheel of your car will increase the degree of contraction (and possibly pain) in the muscles of your lower back, neck, and legs.

A word of encouragement: Loosening up doesn't only happen in the physical body. As you let go of tension in your muscles, you may find that emotional "muscles" are loosened up as well. That may be a welcome relief or it may provide a challenge for you. If you've kept your grief or fear under control with a tight body armor for a long time, such feelings may be unwelcome when they first start to wiggle free. Actually, you are offering yourself a gift with this kind of loosening up. Take it slowly; take all the time you need to befriend your feelings, as we've discussed in Chapter 4: Befriend Your Feelings (page 38). Refer back to that section.

Loosen Up All Over

In order to appreciate wellness, your whole system needs to be relaxed and opened up and flexible. You need to be open enough to receive the energy that breathing and food and movement and light and human communication offer you. It's hard to receive a gift with a closed fist. Once you have a better idea of your patterns of holding or contracting, you can consciously initiate the practice of letting go. In some cases, you may need to visit a health professional who specializes in your particular condition. For instance, TMJ (temporal-mandibular joint) syndrome, a chronically tight condition of the jaw, can be helped with biofeedback training, among other approaches. But for most patterns of tension, self-care is all you need.

See Chapter 3: Breathe for Life (page 32) to learn how to breathe more fully.

See Chapter 29: Put Yourself in the Picture of Health (page 193) for help in creating visualizations.

* USE YOUR BREATH. When you notice tension, consciously direct your breath into that part of the body. Imagine, as you inhale, that the oxygen is flowing freely, in and around the tense spots. Feel it loosening muscles and supplying renewed energy to that area.

* USE VISUAL IMAGERY. When you find your shoulders (or any part of your body) tight, create an image that soothes you. For example, imagine that you are standing under a warm shower that is softening the tough places or washing away the tension; or see yourself floating on a cloud.

* USE SELF-MASSAGE. You don't need to know any fancy massage techniques to release tension in your

body. If your face is contracted with worry or concentration, a few gentle strokes with your fingertips in the tense areas can transform them. When you touch a part of your body consciously and tell it to relax, it often will, immediately.

* USE SELF-TALK. It is possible to alleviate the pain and tension caused by contracted muscles by simply repeating a soothing phrase. "My lower back is loosening and warming," for instance. The talk focuses your attention on the hurting place, and that attention catalyzes the relaxation of the muscles.

* MOVE THE TENSION OUT. Physical exercise is a great way to relieve overall bodily tension. Go for a swim or a brisk walk, or put on some music and dance. Pretend that you are shaking the tension off as you move. You will find that you actually are.

See Chapter 13: Welcome Necessary, Healing Touch—The Gift of Massage (page 92) for more suggestions about self-massage.

Refer back to Chapter 6: Watch Your Words—Avoid Illness Programming (page 52) for suggestions about the use of healing words and phrases.

See Chapter 15: Move for the Health of It—Do Something Aerobic (page 109) for exercise ideas.

11 Find Your Center—Learn to Meditate

Living on planet earth in the twenty-first century is hard on the soul as well as on the body. The stresses that bombard you from all directions, in addition to making you more vulnerable to disease, can leave you feeling unsettled and fragmented—out of touch with what you really want, what you really believe, and ultimately who you really are.

In order to stay happy and healthy, your soul needs nourishment, just as your body does. Many meditation forms are popular today because they are so nourishing. They aid in relaxation, concentration, and an attunement to deeper, more spiritual aspects of your self. Meditation is a process of locating your center of being, your temple of inner wisdom, your truest self, and learning to live, consistently, from that place. It is a way to re-collect your scattered parts. The word "meditation" comes from the Sanskrit word *medha*, which literally means "doing the wisdom."

The more faithfully you listen to the voice within you, the better you will hear what is sounding outside.

DAG HAMMARSKJÖLD

Begin to Meditate

1. Set aside at least ten minutes a day, and eventually longer, in a quiet and private place. (Most meditation forms range in length of practice time from twenty minutes to an hour.)

2. Be prepared to encounter numerous mental distractions. Let them rise and fall or float away like leaves in a moving stream. But don't get washed away with them. Develop an attitude of passive acceptance.

3. Select a centering device. This can be a sound or word or phrase—a mantra—that is repeated. (For example: "One" or "Peace" or a phrase like "There is only love.") Or use a candle or devotional picture to keep your attention focused. You can sing an inspirational song, recite a favorite poem, or use a repetitious bodily movement like swaying or rocking to create a similar centering focus. Concentrating on the breath as it rises and falls or simply counting breaths are other common forms of centering.

4. With extraneous thoughts now in the background, the body and mind are free to rest deeply. For some people, this naturally evolves into a time of wordless gratitude. Others find they more clearly hear or perceive their intuition or inner voice.

5. Keep bringing your attention back to your center. As your mind wanders, and it always will, imagine that you are taking it gently by the hand and leading it back—the way you might lead an exuberant child back to the sidewalk on the way to school. Let gentleness be the guiding principle.

The practice of meditation . . . involves an appreciation of basic, unconditional goodness and a stance of gentleness and fearlessness in dealing with ourselves and our world. In other words, we can maintain our dignity in both illness and health.

Dr. Mitchell Levy

6. Use resources as you need them. There are many books available that will teach you simple meditation practices. In many cities there are groups devoted to teaching and practicing meditation techniques. Energy is greatly intensified when meditation is done with a group. You will be amazed at how many people privately practice some form of personal spiritual practice like meditation. Start asking and listen to what people have to say.

Finding a center, a home, a place of balance within makes almost anything easier to face. The universe, from this perspective, seems friendly, and your place in it feels blessed. Since your life energy emanates from your center, being there regularly means being in greater harmony with yourself, your brothers and sisters, and the cosmos.

To love is to approach each other center to center.

PIERRE TEILHARD DE CHARDIN

Finding Center

People commonly speak of being "off center," meaning imbalanced in some way. Finding a center within your body, a place you can attend to when you are stressed or upset and need to draw your fragmented parts back together, can be helpful. Where would you locate your center? Unsure? Try one or more of these suggestions:

1. If you imagine that your soul exists in your body, where would it be? Touch that place now.

2. Imagine that your body is a building with a hidden chamber located somewhere within it. In that chamber you meet your inner wisdom or guide. This is a place in which no lies can exist. Where is that place?

3. Imagine that you want to balance your physical body. Where is the fulcrum, the point of contact at which you will balance?

4. Take a few slow and very deep breaths. From what place does the breath originate? What place does the deepest breath reach?

5. Say "I am me" several times as you point to yourself. Where do you point? Which place feels truest?

You may have found several different places that felt like your center, your internal home. Decide which one is your favorite for now and experiment with it for at least a week before you try out another one. Use that place within as a point of focus that you can return to even in the midst of chaotic activity. Meditation will

See Chapter 25: Cultivate Sanity through Silence (page 175) for ways to create and enjoy a more quiet environment.

become a way of life, not just something you do for a set time every day. This form of self-remembering is a powerful means of heightening your awareness of your life, reducing stress, altering the way in which you see the world, and consequently enhancing your overall health and wellness.

12 Drink More Water—And Other Healthy Uses of H_2O

If you could accurately assess your body's need for water, you'd probably find that you are at least two quarts low.

ANONYMOUS

All humans come from the water—evolving from the creatures of the sea, bathing in the uterus of the mother. Everyone is primarily made of water, which accounts for about 70 percent of our overall body weight.

Water is essential to balanced health. The body relies on it for digestion, cooling, elimination, and the circulation of nutrients to every cell. Low-level dehydration is commonplace, and many people are unaware when this occurs since they do not feel thirsty. So drink up! Eight big glasses of clear pure water a day is a good recommendation to follow. Don't assume that you are getting enough water from the foods you eat and the beverages you consume. Many water-based beverages, like coffee and soft drinks, contain caffeine and sugar, which actually have a dehydrating effect. More water is required to aid in their digestion and metabolism.

Unless your system is flushed regularly from the inside out, toxins from food and air will accumulate in fat cells (everyone has them), muscles, and joints, causing pain and stiffness and various health problems. Most kidney stones, for instance, consist of urates, phosphates, oxalates, and other wastes that have crystallized from urine that was too concentrated to be excreted as dissolved solids. To protect against this kind of accretion, drink lots of water. Constipation and headaches are often the result of insufficient water in your system. If your feces are hard and small, and sink rather than float, this may also indicate that there is not enough water in your diet.

Drinking plenty of water also aids in maintaining your ideal weight, since water provides oral gratification and gives you a temporary sense of fullness. Some types of overeating may be the body's way of compensating for the lack of water it craves.

Many urban water supplies contain industrial pollutants such as lead, asbestos, and mercury, as well as agricultural chemical pollutants from aquifer contamination and surface water runoff. These accumulate in the body over time. Consider using bottled spring water that has been tested by an independent laboratory (call or write the bottling company), or attaching a high-quality filter to your spigot.

Other Ways to Use Water for Better Health

Now that you consider water to be a necessary part of your diet and a source of inner cleansing, look at some of the ways that it can refresh, cleanse, and heal you from without.

Important: Those with a history of heart disease or high blood pressure should check with a health professional before using the water treatments suggested.

* SHOWERS. Alternate hot and cold water to aid circulation. Showers are also great for washing away the accumulated tension and worries of the day as they relax your body and break up the psychic residue left by the negativity of others with whom you have interacted during the day.

* BATHS. Nothing tops a bath to help alleviate muscle soreness. If your bath is warm enough to make you sweat a bit, it is providing the added benefit of releasing wastes through the steam-opened pores of your skin. For relaxation, fill a tub with comfortably hot water and add a few drops of mild bath oil to moisturize

your skin, or add your favorite scented oil. Light a candle. Burn some incense if you like. Have a glass of juice. Play some soft, slow music. Nurture yourself.

* SWIMMING. Regular swimming is a great form of aerobic exercise. Or you can exercise in water to achieve similar benefits. Whether you know how to swim or not, it is therapeutic just to get in the shallow water and splash out your frustrations or problems. Be a child again—play!

* SWEATING (in a sauna, steam bath, or sweat lodge) or SOAKING (in a spa, hot tub, or mineral springs). These ancient remedies for stress and pain are as valuable today as they have been for centuries. If you can't get to a spa, soaking your feet in the bathtub or a basin at home is a simple way to enjoy and heal yourself.

* HOT COMPRESSES. Grate some fresh gingerroot and wrap it in cheesecloth. Place the bundle in a large pot of water. Heat the water, but do not let it boil. Turn off the heat and soak a towel in the water. Carefully remove the towel; let it cool until it is comfortable enough to handle, then wring it out. Apply the towel to any ailing body part. Leave it on until the heat is exhausted. Then do it again.

* RITUALS. Compose a ceremony in which you use water to symbolically cleanse your body, mind, and soul

from illness, darkness, "sin," and painful memories. This is a beautiful way to love yourself.

Go get yourself a big glass of water right now. Drink it slowly and experience it with all your senses.

13 Welcome Necessary, Healing Touch—The Gift of Massage

The skin is the largest organ of your body and accounts for almost one-fifth of your total body weight. The skin is constantly growing and changing in sensitivity as it performs its many functions: protection, sensation, temperature regulation, excretion, respiration, and the metabolism and storage of fat.

Touch is the first sense to develop in a newborn. As an infant takes her first breath, she reaches out to learn what her new world is all about. Sensory receptors located in the skin start picking up enormous quantities of information and sending them to the brain. Pressure, temperature, pleasure, pain—each stimulus carries a message about the environment. Each one adds another tidbit to the infant's store of experience.

For a baby to develop normally, it is essential that she be touched, physically handled. When touching is denied or severely restricted, an infant may actually die. Thousands of children in U.S. foundling homes (orphanages for the very young) died until, in the late 1920s, this connection between touch and life was understood and remedied. Adults who were deprived of physical stroking in childhood often adopt compulsive, destructive habits such as nailbiting, overeating, or smoking. There is some speculation that violent behavior may also be a result of touch deprivation in early childhood. Cross-cultural and laboratory research both reveal a strong association between early child-care practices and later violent behavior. The child who receives a great deal of attention, whose every need is promptly met, becomes a gentle, cooperative, nonaggressive adult. The child who receives intermittent attention often becomes a selfish, uncooperative, depressed, or aggressive adult.

Yet few adults appreciate how valuable touch can be. Many adults actually avoid bodily contact. If they weren't touched with care and nurturance as children, they may view touching with suspicion and fear. Many people even fear their own bodies and are reluctant to touch or massage themselves. They are not comfortable with their own skin. Others were taught long ago that touching themselves was sinful, and that vestige of fear remains, especially in sexual expression. Because of the cultural connection between touch and sex, some people are loath to touch others except in formal handshakes, not wanting their actions to be misjudged. Those who are afraid to touch or be touched deprive themselves of a powerful source of nurturance and healing. In fact, when they are depressed or anxious, they may show an even greater tendency to withdraw from the very things that would help them feel better—a reassuring touch, a sympathetic hug, a healing massage.

There is a growing acceptance of therapeutic massage within the medical profession. In the 1970s, at the New York University Medical Center, Dolores Krieger, PhD, RN, conducted a study to determine the value of what she called "therapeutic touch." One group of patients received regular care; another group received a simple form of touch from their nurses, similar to the laying on of hands, twice a day. Within one day, significant results were realized. The patients who were touched had increased blood hemoglobin levels (hemoglobin, which is found in the red blood cells, carries oxygen from the lungs to the other body tissues), which aided their recovery. The control group of patients showed no change in this aspect. In other test cases, Krieger verified the value of therapeutic touch in accelerating the healing process. Patients suffering stress-related diseases who experienced this form of touch consistently report feeling profound relaxation and an alleviation of pain and other symptoms, such as nausea, poor circulation, and tachycardia (excessively rapid heartbeat).

As a form of nurturance and rebalancing, and as an aid to healing, massage is hard to beat. Besides, it's nonfattening, and if you do it yourself, it's free. Some positive results of massage include:

* relief of pain and tension
* improved muscle tone
* a healthy complexion
* the release of emotional blocks caused by trauma and repression
* increased blood flow and electrical energy to "wake up" your tired body parts
* pleasure
* a general balancing of right and left, and upper and lower parts of your body

Begin with Self-Massage

Self-massage is a type of self-care—a way to heal, increase self-awareness, and build self-appreciation. Besides, it feels great and it's easy to do. You simply put your hands on your body and start moving them. Lotions, special techniques, and formal training can certainly enhance the experience, but they can also lead you to believe that you need them to do massage "right." Not true. As you massage yourself, listen with your hands and let them accept feedback from your body and respond accordingly. The more you can quiet the chatter and judgment in your mind and allow your hands to move intuitively, the more creative, relaxed, and enjoyable the results will be.

See Chapter 2: Inhabit Your Body and Love It (page 26) to learn more about appreciating your body.

Try a Head Massage

1. Remove any glasses or contact lenses and turn down any bright lights. Rub your hands together to warm them. Slightly cup your palms, fingers together, and place them on your face. Hold them there for thirty seconds or so while you relax.

2. When ready, let your hands move over your face in a variety of slow or rhythmic movements, as you like: Make circular moves with fingertips, follow the contours

of your face with finger pressure, knead your skin, and so on. Take your time.

3. Move your fingertips onto your skull and through your hair. Press all over. Try tapping or rubbing your scalp, or even grasping and firmly pulling your hair for additional stimulation. Explore other options for yourself. Be creative.

4. Stroke your head and face smoothly and gently all over, soothing your eyes, ears, lips, and throat. Say nice things to yourself as you do this.

5. Using your fingertips, massage your gums by feeling them through your cheeks.

6. Gently and sensuously wash your face, or apply warm towels to it. Splash your face with cold water to conclude, and apply some natural oil or lotion for a moisture treatment.

And a Foot Massage

The rubbing of tired feet is an age-old practice. In Oriental medicine, body energy, or *chi,* is believed to flow lengthwise along energy meridians that end in our feet. Several contemporary therapeutic approaches, like zone therapy and foot reflexology, suggest that there are points on your feet that correspond to every part of your body, such as endocrine glands or the spinal column. Thus working on your feet is comparable to massaging your entire body. Practitioners of foot reflexology believe that pressure or massage to the feet can break up energy blockages and recharge the corresponding segment of your body. While many of these claims are not yet fully scientifically verified, the value of foot massage as a simple, loving, and therefore healing tool is undisputed by anyone who has ever received one.

1. Position yourself so you can comfortably hold one of your feet in both hands.

2. Using massage oil or lotion, if you wish, rub your feet and ankles all over. Massage your heel, the areas between your toes, the top as well as the bottom of your foot, and your arch. Generally, wake your foot up.

3. With specific pressure from your thumb pad or the knuckle of your index finger, explore your toes and feet

for areas of soreness and sensitivity. Gently massage those areas, using a smooth, circular motion for fifteen seconds or less. Then move on to another area.

4. When you are finished, rub your foot all over as if you were smoothing the skin. Stretch your toes and rotate your ankle. Then begin on your other foot.

Massage for Pain Relief

While severe or long-term pain should always be checked out by a health professional, you can help yourself with everyday pains and aches. If you can reach the part your body that is in pain, you may be able to relieve the ache. Using both hands if possible, cup them slightly and lay them over the painful area. Now begin to breathe slowly and deeply. Imagine that you are breathing warmth and energy through your hands into your body at that point. Imagine that this warmth and energy flows into you through the top of your head and flows out through your hands. Imagine the pain and tension melting away under your hands.

Keep your hands in the same position until you feel a shift in your overall level of relaxation or a lessening in the degree of pain.

Use Massage with Others Too

All of the exercises suggested above can be done with a partner. Consider sharing the gift of touch with another person and allowing yourself to receive this gift in return. Again, it isn't necessary to have formal training. Your intention to offer comfort or relief is all you need to use a healing touch.

The arrival of a good clown exercises more beneficial influence upon the health of a town than twenty asses laden with drugs.

THOMAS SYDENHAM,
seventeenth-century physician

14 Lighten Up with Humor, Play, and Pleasure

The process of becoming healthier can be presented as such serious business that you lose much of the humor and joy of living that characterize wellbeing. Many books about health are filled with predictions of dire consequences for failure to follow particular methods, horror stories of what certain foods or lack of foods can do, or warnings about the cancer-causing qualities of everything. It's enough to make you crazy!

Recent studies indicate that humor is an effective stress reducer and that it may actually increase antibody production, which means a stronger immune system. In 1964, Norman Cousins, then editor of *Saturday Review,* helped to heal himself from a life-threatening disease through a regimen of vitamin C, renewed self-responsibility, and humor. His reading of several classic books on the subject of stress convinced him that disease was fostered by chemical changes in the body produced by emotions such as anger and fear. He wondered whether an antidote of hope, love, laughter, and the will to live would have the opposite effect. Encouraged by watching Marx Brothers movies and *Candid Camera* TV sequences, reading humorous books and stories, and listening to jokes, he found that short periods of hearty laughter were enough to induce several hours of painless sleep. Years later, Cousins recommended laughter to others, claiming that this "inner exercising" was beneficial in stimulating breathing, muscular activity, and heart rate.

Worldwide interest continues to grow in establishing the benefits of laughter and humor in health, supported by wide-ranging scientific research. The Humor Project Inc., based in Saratoga Springs, New York, one of many associations dedicated to tickling the funny bone, publishes *Laughing Matters Magazine* in twenty countries, and offers Daily Laffirmations through its Web site, www.humorproject.com.

Raymond Moody Jr., MD, the author of *Laugh after Laugh: The Healing Power of Humor,* has used this

Therapeutic humor is any intervention that promotes health and wellness by stimulating a playful discovery, expression or appreciation of the absurdity or incongruity of life's situations. This intervention may enhance health or be used as a complementary treatment of illness to facilitate healing or coping, whether physical, emotional, cognitive, social, or spiritual.

THE AMERICAN ASSOCIATION OF THERAPEUTIC HUMOR

approach with his patients for many years. Humor works, he claims, because laughter helps take your mind off pain and problems, and catalyzes the basic will to live.

Our favorite comedians are Whoopi Goldberg, George Carlin, Bette Midler, John Candy, Eddie Murphy, Adam Sandler, Lily Tomlin, and Steve Martin.

Take a Seriousness Break Right Now

Look in the mirror and make the wildest, most distorted face you can make. Now make an even wilder one.

Throw away your troubles. Stand up right now. Form your hands into fists and bring them together at the center of your chest. Raise your elbows on a line with your fists. Thrust your shoulders and elbows back sharply, as if you are trying to shake something off your back and shoulders. After the thrust, let your fists come together again at the level of your chest, and thrust your shoulders and elbows back again. Do this six to eight times in rapid succession, saying "get off my back" each time you thrust back. Release whatever is burdening you.

It takes a long time to become young.

PABLO PICASSO

Read the comics in today's paper. Forget the front page for a while.

Put on a comedy video, if you have one. Cue it up to your favorite funny part, and play it and replay it several times. Rent a few comedy tapes or go to a light, entertaining movie. Do this regularly.

Collect jokes. Ask anyone around you for a joke or two. Get on an e-mail joke-mailing list. Call a friend and have them tell you a joke, even if they know you've heard it before. Now you share one with them. Get silly!

Watch young children at play. Note the spontaneity and sheer delight that often characterizes their activities.

Remember laughing so hard that your stomach hurt? Can you recall what provoked that? Let yourself feel it again.

Redefining Play

Play is an essential component of wellness. It is necessary to keep the fun-loving part of yourself alive, nurtured, and happy. The dictionary defines play as recreation. Re-creation! So, in the fullest sense of the term, it means to make new, to vitalize again, to inspire with life and energy. When you give yourself time to play you give yourself new life.

What words do you associate with play? Are they active words, like *silliness, craziness, sports, games, excitement?* Perhaps one of the reasons people don't play more is that they have accepted a very narrow definition of play. Maybe they've looked around at what society tells them is "fun" to do and found that it wasn't.

Imagine the world without pleasure. Life would appear colorless and humorless, a baby's smile would go unappreciated. Foods would be tasteless. The genius of a Bach concerto would fall on deaf ears. Feelings like joy, thrills, delights, ecstasy, elation, and happiness would disappear. The company of others would bring no comfort or joy. The touch of a mother would no longer soothe, and a lover could not arouse. Interest in sex and procreation would dry up. The next generation would await unborn.

Ornstein and Sobel,
Healthy Pleasures

Consider that play can also be described as *absorbing, fascinating, peaceful, flowing, restful*—that it needn't be highly organized or competitive. Perhaps you have forgotten the natural play of your childhood, when you could lose yourself in exploring rocks, making a fantasy realm out of a chair and a sheet, or singing for your own amusement.

See Chapter 3: Breathe for Life (page 32), Chapter 9: Stretch Yourself (page 70), Chapter 11: Find Your Center—Learn to Meditate (page 83), Chapter 15: Move for the Health of It—Do Something Aerobic (page 109), and Chapter 16: Develop Personal Nutritional Awareness (page 119) for additional ways to slow down and enjoy your life.

It is easy to get caught up in the frenzy of filling every minute of your working hours with meaningful business. But this becomes a self-defeating strategy when it flows into your leisure time as well. The fear of "wasting" time has become an obsession for many, so they end up on a fast track of play.

Teenagers suggest that you "chill out," or "relax, dude." These admonitions are important as you approach play. Please don't use any of the ideas here to burden yourself with increased demands on your time and energy. Perhaps it's time to just do nothing for some part of each day. Slowing down long enough to receive the simple pleasures that are all around you is one of the most effective ways to deepen your enjoyment of life and thereby enhance your overall health.

What's Your Pleasure?

What does play mean to you? Is there enough fun in your life? Enough time for simply fooling around? You will find it easier to begin exploring this subject by making a Non-pleasure List of things that aren't fun or playful or enjoyable for you. Things like skydiving, or shopping for clothes, or running. You may even get a laugh or two out of making the list. Once that list is out of the way, you may be inspired to make a Pleasure List of what *is* fun for you—like checking out garage sales, going out for breakfast with a friend, or taking a sauna.

Go through your Pleasure List and indicate the last time you remember doing each of these activities. Is there one item on your list that you could do today? One that you will put on your schedule for this week or next? Many people find it helpful to actually put the date on their calendar, scheduling in times for doing something fun or for just doing nothing.

We stake our lives on our purposeful programs and projects, our serious jobs and endeavors. But doesn't the really important part of our life unfold "after hours"—singing and dancing, music and painting, prayer and lovemaking, or just fooling around?

FR. WILLIAM MCNAMARA

PART III
taking action

*

IF YOUR PROGRESS THROUGH THIS BOOK has been like a leisurely hike along the foothills, consider that you have now reached the base of the mountain. The path of ascent stretches before you, sometimes rocky, sometimes steep. In Part III you will encounter information, exercises, and choices that will demand more of a commitment to making wellness a way of life rather than a hobby or weekend diversion. You will have to decide that you are going to stay on course. When you decide to alter your diet, for instance, results may not be immediately apparent. In fact, you may actually go through a period of feeling worse before you start to feel better, since your body will have to cope with the symptoms of withdrawal from sugar and other addictive substances.

We suggest that you start with the areas that address your most pressing concern—such as nutrition, exercise, relationships, or communication—and that you use the resources suggested at the end of the book to deepen your self-understanding. Work on just one area for at least several weeks before moving on to another area. Refer back to Part I and Part II, especially to those areas that will support you as your start taking action.

PART III ADDRESSES:

* aerobic exercise
* nutritional awareness
* dietary change
* commonsense safety measures
* building friendships
* improved listening skills for improved communications
* assertiveness training
* creating a healthier work environment
* cleaning up your environment

15 Move for the Health of It—Do Something Aerobic

Everything inside your body is moving. Your heart pumps, blood flows, lungs expand and contract, eyes roll, eardrums vibrate, atoms dance, and neurons fire. As a result, you walk, reach out and touch the world around you, stretch yourself, and dance. Movement is a sign of life. Seriously inhibit the movement of limbs and organs, and you encourage illness. Stop motion altogether and you are dead. Allow yourself to move as fully as possible both within and without, and you realize wellness.

The labor of the human body is rapidly being engineered out of working life.

JOHN F. KENNEDY

Since the Industrial Revolution, life has changed dramatically. People no longer chop wood and carry water. Earning a livelihood generally involves sitting for long hours at a computer terminal or in an automobile, or standing behind a counter or at an assembly line. With rare exception, people's requirements to move vigorously are few. Cars, buses, trains, planes, telephones, computers, overnight parcels, and fax machines do it for them.

Is the U.S. leading the Western world into an international culture of overweight couch potatoes?

Statistics indicate that the average eighth grader in the U.S. can't pass a minimal fitness test, and many people think nothing about driving their car to a destination a few blocks away instead of walking. Heart disease is the leading cause of death in most developed countries, and lack of exercise is one of its primary risk factors.

Without exercise at all, as happens when you are confined to bed, the muscles lose 15 percent of their strength for every week of inactivity. So if you lead a sedentary life, chances are that your muscles are weak and therefore more injury prone. But the good news is that this strength can be regained, and the heart can be reconditioned. The body is amazingly resilient. Even years of neglect can be compensated for by a regular program of aerobic physical exercise.

Not Just Jogging

Aerobics is any system of conditioning exercises that increases heart and breathing rates for a sustained period and thus increases the flow of oxygen and blood to all parts of the body. To be effective, the exercise must raise the pulse rate to a certain level (see the following chart) and keep it at that level for not less than twenty minutes. (Note: People who are not in good physical condition should start out with ten minutes at the minimum heart rate and build to twenty minutes at the maximum heart rate.)

Aerobic conditioning benefits the body in many ways. It will decrease intramuscular fat and increase lean muscle, leading to a firmer, stronger body. Aerobic exercise improves circulation; a trained heart is a more efficient pump and therefore doesn't have to work so hard. This lowered heart rate preserves the heart and lessens its chance of fatiguing prematurely. Aerobics improves absorption and utilization of food; provides overall increases in energy and stamina; encourages more restful sleep; and decreases dependence on addictive substances such as alcohol, drugs, and tobacco. Most exercisers report a decrease in nervous tension and depression. And it is now known that exercise causes the release of certain brain chemicals (endorphins and enkephalins) that increase an overall sense of wellbeing.

If you are not in the habit of exercising regularly, you may hear the word "aerobics," and immediately see visions of thin, tight bodies in coordinated workout gear, or think with dread about running. Don't be discouraged. A wellness approach to exercise is not that limited.

Heart Rates

Age	*Minimum HR*	*Maximum HR*
20	120	160
22	119	158
24	118	157
26	116	155
28	115	154
30	114	152
32	113	150
34	112	149
36	110	147
38	109	146
40	108	144
45	105	140
50	102	136
55	99	132
60	96	128
65	93	124
70	90	120
75	87	116
80	84	112

Design Your Own Program

Every body is different, and every psyche is different too. If you have resisted exercise in the past but know that it's time for a change, it is especially important that you design a program you can live with and stay with—a gentle, step-by-step program that will appeal to your fun-loving inner child or provide companionship or quiet time alone, depending on your needs and desires. Jogging or running are definitely not the only ways to move your body. Consider these other forms of aerobic exercise:

* dancing of all kinds (even ballroom dancing can elevate the heart rate)
* swimming and other water programs, including aerobics for nonswimmers
* walking, walking, walking, walking, walking
* hiking and climbing
* bicycling
* skipping, jumping rope, or jumping on a trampoline
* calisthenics and weight training
* rowing
* tennis and other ball sports
* using indoor equipment like stationary bikes, treadmills, or rowing machines

Choose one or more forms of aerobic exercise that you think you will enjoy and try them out. You know which exercise form you are more likely to stay with. Avoid setting yourself up for failure and disappointment by forcing yourself to be brave or strong about your exercise. Taking a vigorous walk around your block every day is infinitely more beneficial than dreaming about doing a triathlon.

But if the dance of the run isn't fun
then discover another dance
because without fun
the good of the run
is undone
and a suffering runner
always quits
sooner or later.

FRED ROHE,
The Zen of Running

* DON'T BE IN A HURRY. It takes time to recondition your heart. Before starting a program, we recommend a physical exam and an EKG, especially if you are over forty. Make realistic goals for yourself and reward every effort. Promise yourself small, healthy treats for accomplishing, or even approximating, your goals.

* REGULAR EXERCISE IS IMPERATIVE. Three times a week, your exercise should maintain your training pulse rate for at least fifteen minutes. (See the preceding chart.) Block out exercise time in your weekly calendar. Call a friend and exercise together. Keep a daily log of your progress. Do anything and everything that will keep you moving.

* ALWAYS START YOUR EXERCISE WITH WARM-UPS, and complete it with a cooling-down period that includes some stretching.

* Avoid imitation. Learn from the pros but don't hold yourself back by comparing yourself with them. Treasure your own uniqueness. And deal cautiously with competition—even if it's with yourself. Let yourself lose, or win, graciously.

* Follow spontaneous impulses and use every means available to stay inspired. When the urge to move arises, seize it. Close the office door and jump rope, or hang up the phone and run around the house.

* Breathe. Inhale as your movements expand, exhale as they contract or move back to center. You are overexerting if you can't talk comfortably as you exercise, or if your heart rate is not back to 120, or less, five minutes after completing your exercise. Normal breathing should return within ten minutes after exertion.

* If pain starts, stop. Honor your body's natural warning system, especially in the beginning. Danger signs that you should stop exercising include faintness, dizziness, nausea, tightness or pain in the chest, severe shortness of breath, or loss of muscle control.

* Whatever you're doing—dance it. Practice moving from the inside out, smoothly, as if you were dancing, and the sense of rightness and connectedness that follows will make exercising a pleasant experience.

When exercising outdoors, dance with the earth as you move on it.

Two Exercise Breaks

* TAKE A WALK. Walk briskly for at least ten to fifteen minutes. Start out at the rate of approximately three miles (five kilometers) per hour. Move your whole body. Don't be embarrassed to swing your arms as you walk; this will create a massaging action on the lymph glands in your armpits and stimulate the natural detoxifying function of these glands. Enjoy looking around at your environment as you walk along. Listen to the birds and smell the flowers.

Build up the length of time you spend walking. Increase it by five minutes a week until you can easily walk two miles in thirty-five minutes if you are a woman, and in twenty-eight minutes if you are a man. What could be a simpler way to start your aerobic conditioning than to do something you've been doing all your life? People are increasingly turning to walking as their preferred form of exercise because it is so much easier on the legs than running, and because there is no need for special equipment except a comfortable pair of walking shoes.

* JOIN THE DANCE. You may be surprised at how easy and joyful movement can be. The following exercise gets you dancing in a way that is energizing and fun. Read the directions over once or twice before you begin so you won't have to stop once the movement starts. Here's what to do:

1. Play a recording of a slow, gentle piece of music, or tune your radio to a classical or easy listening station. Then close your eyes and simply listen to the music for a few minutes. Breathe it in.

2. Begin to move by directing your attention to your right hand, and start to tap or stretch those fingers in any way that the music suggests. Allow the movement to extend, encompassing your wrist as well. Keep doing this simple movement for a while. Then direct your attention to the left hand and do the same. Imagine that you are directing an orchestra, or splashing in water, or molding a piece of clay to represent what you are hearing. Play with the sound. Next, engage your right arm, and then your left, allowing yourself to move from your shoulders to the tips of your fingers. How many different ways can you find to

bend them, to position them, to move them in unison or in opposition?

3. Keep your arms and hands going, doing whatever they want to, as you now pay attention to your head. Let the music direct it. Conduct the symphony with a baton that extends from the center of your forehead, from the crown, from your chin.

4. Your upper body now wants to get into the act. Concentrate on your middle section. Allow yourself to bend and sway from the waist in any way that feels good. Pretend that your whole body consists of the area from your waist to your head; forget the rest. Let your hips and pelvis join in the movement only when you are ready for them. Careful here; they will want to take over.

5. Imagine yourself as a tree in the wind. Your roots are firm. Only your branches and upper trunk sway. Be a fettered bird wanting to escape, but restrained by a silver thread. Fantasize that you are a belly dancer, write your name with an imaginary pencil that extends from your left hip. Write "I love you" with the imaginary pencil.

6. Unlock your knees and move your legs without lifting your feet. Challenge yourself with how many ways you can direct your legs, ways that you never tried before. Pretend that you are scientifically cataloguing all the possible combinations of movement that legs can make. Keep your feet still until you can't stand it a minute longer. Go within yourself and note what every part of your body feels like. Imagine your blood cells dancing, your oxygen dancing, and your energy dancing.

7. Now let go completely and allow yourself to move totally—head, arms, belly, pelvis, legs, feet. Surprise! Want another exercise? Try a different, perhaps more active, piece of music.

16 Develop Personal Nutritional Awareness

Food and nutrition are enormously popular subjects today. Food companies are climbing on the bandwagon, offering products that are vitamin enriched, low in salt, high in fiber, or caffeine or cholesterol free. People are preoccupied with cutting down on fat and cholesterol. They are also inclined, because of their high-speed lifestyles, to eat more fast foods, which are notoriously high in both fat and cholesterol. The numerous popular diets and the growing body of nutritional information confuse many people. Since even the experts often disagree among themselves, it's no wonder that nutrition has become almost as controversial as religion or politics.

In the 1960s, the pioneering work of Roger J. Williams, PhD, introduced the concept of biochemical individuality, which said that each person has unique biochemical needs that can only be met by a personalized balance of nutrients. His work ushered in the era of individual nutritional analyses, metabolic profiles, personalized health plans, and specially designed diets (such as eating for your blood type or your ayurvedic type). While such workups may be valuable, unless they rest on a foundation of self-understanding, they become one more way of relinquishing your wellbeing to the control of others. You need to develop an awareness of your own nutritional needs and to understand your own relationship to foods. You can become a partner with the experts, using the information they supply to supplement what you know about yourself. Then you can decide what makes nutritional sense for you.

In Chapter 2: Inhabit Your Body and Love It (page 26) we spoke generally of tuning in to your body's feedback system, of listening to and inhabiting your body. What follows builds on these concepts, applying this awareness specifically to food and eating habits. We suggest that you review Chapter 2 before proceeding.

Developing awareness of your body and its nutritional needs means that you observe—with honesty, sensitivity, and thoroughness—what types and quantities of food and what eating environments support your overall wellbeing, and which don't. When you eat so quickly that you don't have time to savor your food, when you use food to soothe emotional pain, or when you get in the habit of overeating, you soon lose awareness of what food is doing for you. As you sharpen your ability to understand what your body is telling you about its relationship to food, you reinforce the conscious lifestyle that you have chosen. This type of awareness is an effective way of breaking the dieting habit forever. Instead of waging war with your body, you form an alliance with it, feeding it what it really wants and needs in order to support you.

Taking Stock

These exercises that follow will help you sharpen your self-awareness, and may point out some areas that need more attention to support your overall health.

A Nutrition Journal

A NUTRITION JOURNAL CAN BE USED AS A:

* personal record of your body's responses to the foods you eat
* balance sheet to observe the kinds of raw materials and fuels with which you supply your body
* place to keep special recipes
* diet notebook for weight gain and/or loss
* record of your feelings and resolutions

1. Find out what you are eating, when, and how the food makes you feel by keeping a Nutritional Journal for a week or more. Record anything that you learn about your relationship to food and use this knowledge, when you're ready, to design a simpler and healthier diet for yourself.

2. Pause for a moment and become aware of how hungry your body feels. Ask yourself, on a scale of 1 to 10, where 1 = fainting from hunger and 10 = overstuffed, just how hungry you are now. Do this several times during the day to heighten your self-awareness and to get in the habit of eating only when your hunger score is 5 or less. Learn to distinguish between stomach hunger and mouth hunger. Mouth hunger is usually experienced in the jaws, tongue, teeth, and gums—which want to chew on or be stimulated by something—or in a salivary reaction prompted by the sight of food or food cues, such as a restaurant sign or images of eating on TV. Mouth hunger often indicates a need for attention, affection, pain relief, or security of some sort.

3. Observe bodily signs that indicate imbalances in your diet. Look at your tongue, for instance. If it is

frequently discolored or coated, or if you consistently have bad breath or a sour taste in your mouth, you need a change of diet. The health of your gums and teeth are indicators both of good dental care and of a healthy diet. Teeth can become discolored from caffeine and nicotine, and eating foods with lots of sugar can cause cavities. Fingernails that split may mean that your body is not assimilating protein properly. Read your bowel movements for signs of a poor diet. If stools are hard to pass and dark, and sink rather than float, dietary change is indicated. Many processed foods, like white flour products, are slow to move through the intestines. Eating foods with a high fiber content, adding a moderate amount of oil (such as flax [always uncooked], olive, or canola) to your diet, and drinking lots of water will speed intestinal transit time, lowering your risk of colon or intestinal cancer and improving your health in general.

4. Consider headaches as loud and clear messages that something is amiss. Frequently they are indicative of stress, but they are also associated with a host of dietary problems, such as excessive alcohol consumption, reactions to caffeine, undereating or overeating in general, and blood sugar imbalances.

A Nutrition Journal

For example:

Subject under Consideration

BREAKFAST

Day/Time

MONDAY, 3/22, 9:00 A.M.

Breakfast Foods

2 EGGS

BACON—2 STRIPS

TOAST—2 PIECES

BUTTER AND JAM

COFFEE—2 CUPS

Immediate Effects/Later Effects

LEFT THE TABLE FEELING STUFFED. TOO MUCH FOOD. GENERALLY GOOD DAY. NOT HUNGRY UNTIL 3:00 P.M.

Reflections:

Resolutions:

5. Do you experience frequent indigestion? Listening to your body means carefully noting how you feel after eating certain foods. Indigestion is not normal. If you get up from the table or wake up in the morning feeling nauseated, bloated, heavy, or achy, it's time for a change of menu or an adjustment to the quantity of food you consume.

6. Do you have difficulty sleeping? Try to recall what food or drink you consumed in the hours before retiring. Many people find that heavy foods (like pizza), caffeine drinks, or chocolate and other sweets interfere with their ability to fall asleep quickly and stay asleep.

Then What?

Experiment with different foods and different ways of eating. Stay with each experiment long enough to really experience its effects. Add a new food to your diet or stop eating a particular food for a while. Try eating your heaviest meal in the middle of the day instead of evening, or abstain from food for three to four hours before going to bed. Within a few days (or up to a week or two), small dietary changes may result in positive health benefits like greater energy, mental clarity, or better digestion. Be aware that even if the change is a positive one it may feel difficult or uncomfortable, like when we challenge an addiction (caffeine or sugar) or an old habit (overeating). If you aren't sure whether a dietary change is working for you, consult with your doctor or health-care professional.

Educate yourself about nutrition. Read. Talk to your health professionals or those who exemplify healthiness for you, and go on to the next chapter.

17 Learn Ten Basics about Food

This book doesn't prescribe a single system that everyone can or should follow. That would undermine its underlying premise of making your own choices. However, since we strongly advocate eating well for living well, some consideration of the components of sound nutritional practice is needed if you are to develop a diet that will truly support your wellbeing. Although a mass of conflicting data surrounds this subject, certain recommendations are almost universally accepted, and these warrant your attention.

Nutrition Basics

* CHOOSE YOUR FOOD BASED ON ITS LIFE FORCE. Doesn't it make sense that the less your foods are processed the more their essential nutrients will be available for use? When you overcook fruits and vegetables, for example, they lose many of their enzymes, vitamins, and minerals. When you eat foods that have been grown in devitalized soil, food that has been genetically engineered, or fruits and vegetables that have been sprayed with poisonous chemicals and then waxed to look good on the shelf, you are multiplying your health risks. Decreasing your consumption of highly processed foods, especially those that contain additives and preservatives, is one simple step in support of commonsense nutrition. Over time, these food additives take a cumulative toll on your liver, which must break down, detoxify, and excrete or store the unusable substances found in processed foods. Many products (like rice or bread, for example) are "enriched" with vitamins and minerals because they have been so devitalized in their preparation. Develop your taste for simple, lively food. Shop for organically grown produce whenever possible. Enjoy steamed or fresh veggies and fruits in all their wondrous forms.

Eat more fruits and vegetables, five or more servings a day. These foods contain vitamins and minerals in their natural form as well as fiber, which markedly reduces the risk of bowel cancer and other diseases of the intestines. Fruits and vegetables, and other plant foods that have phytochemicals, aid the body in its defense against illness. "Phyto" means "plant," and phytochemicals are those functional components found in plant foods that are responsible for a plant's color, aroma, and flavor, and for protecting the plant from disease. Chlorophyll and beta-carotene are two examples among hundreds, maybe thousands, of phytochemicals that are currently being researched, and more are still being discovered. These wondrous substances are contained in micro amounts in all plant foods. When we ingest them, they impact specific life functions, such as strengthening the immune system or aiding in the production of hormones.

As you increase your consumption of fruits and vegetables, remember to treat yourself to a whole palette of colors to eat from. Look to the sea for vegetables rich in trace minerals that have been lost from our depleted soils. More and more Americans are developing a taste for sea vegetables such as nori, dulse, and wakame.

* EAT FOODS THAT ARE RICH IN THE ANTIOXIDANT PHYTOCHEMICALS THAT ABSORB FREE RADICALS (unpaired electrons produced in various natural and artificial processes, such as cooking with fats and oils). Free radicals encourage peroxidation in the body (which destroys cell walls) and have been linked to cancer, premature aging, degenerative diseases, and many conditions of the hormone systems. Well-known antioxidants like vitamins A, E, C, the mineral selenium, and the enzyme CoQ_{10}—all of which are found in various vegetables, grains, and nuts—actually slow down the aging process and strengthen the immune system.

* EAT WHOLE GRAINS. Brown rice, and other varieties of rice, and grains like wheat, millet, buckwheat, barley, and corn have been the staple foods of people around the world for ages. The complex carbohydrates (starch) found in whole grains make them an excellent source of body fuel, and the natural fibers in grains assist the process of elimination, acting as a preventative to bowel cancer and other intestinal diseases. Brown rice is one of nature's most perfect foods. The USDA Food Pyramid that has replaced many previous systems of nutritional information suggests that grains and foods made from grains (breads, cereals, and pasta)

form the basis of the pyramid, the largest food group, and should be eaten regularly.

* DECREASE YOUR CONSUMPTION OF ANIMAL PRODUCTS. That especially includes red meat, which is unnecessary in a carefully chosen human diet. Diets high in red meat are linked to heart disease and bowel cancer. The chemicals used to fatten and prevent disease in cattle are extremely reactive with the human immune system. The same applies to dairy products, which are highly questionable from a health perspective. Like meat, milk contains high amounts of hormones and other substances fed to cattle to make them more economically productive. Animal milk is a highly allergenic substance for human infants. If you do buy meat and dairy products, educate yourself and search out sources of these products that are produced without homogenization, hormones, or disease-preventing antibiotics.

* REDUCE YOUR OVERALL CONSUMPTION OF SATURATED FATS, particularly animal fats (organic butter is a notable exception), while becoming aware of the "good fats" necessary to good health—like the essential fatty acids found in olive oil, flax oil, and certain fish. A high intake of saturated fats is implicated in heart disease, cancer, and obesity.

* Decrease your consumption of sugar and foods high in added sugar. Eliminating or substantially reducing processed sweets from your diet may not be easy since sugar does provide a quick, short-lived burst of energy that you may have come to rely on. Sugar stresses both the liver and pancreas as they work to counterbalance the effects of the sugar rush. Decreasing your intake of sugar will give your body a chance to rest from such chronic overstress. Less sugar will increase the efficiency of your digestive system, resulting in better physical energy in the long run. Many people who stop the processed-sugar habit find that they have significantly fewer mood swings, headaches, and erratic food cravings. Furthermore, the calories obtained from junk foods create a substitution effect and decrease your appetite for the foods that would give you the nutrients you need.

* Use less salt. Your daily salt requirement is only about one-half gram (about three shakes of a standard salt shaker) and most likely the foods you eat contain more than that even before you salt them. Daily salt consumption in the U.S. ranges from 6 to 18 grams. Salt increases blood pressure in some people. Some research links high salt intake with changes in levels of gastric acid secretion, stomach cancer, and cerebrovascular disease.

* Reduce or completely eliminate your use of caffeine. Caffeine continually overstimulates the adrenals, causing the release of adrenaline into your bloodstream. This is why you feel such a rush from caffeine products. The liver must overcompensate to minimize caffeine's affect on your heart, and this ultimately depletes your energy. When their energy flags, many people simply ingest more caffeine. This erratic pattern is highly stressful on your liver and other organs. Caffeine is clearly an addictive substance, as anyone who has tried to withdraw from it knows.

For those who want the "buzz" that caffeine offers, green tea is a great alternative to other caffeine beverages. Green tea has such a high antioxidant content that it is actually a therapeutic substance.

See Chapter 12: Drink More Water—And Other Healthy Uses of H_2O (page 88) for more information on keeping yourself hydrated.

* Drink plenty of pure water, ideally eight glasses a day. Most people are chronically dehydrated and don't realize it. One of the primary reasons for chronic constipation is a result of failure to drink sufficient quantities of water. That one change is a miracle cure for many people. If you are not sure that your tap water is pure, have it tested. Most tap water contains contaminants; we recommend using a high-quality filter or bottled water.

* Eat consciously. Food has aroma, texture, color, form, temperature, and weight, both on your plate and in your mouth. Don't miss it. Somebody prepared the food you are eating. Somebody worked to purchase it. Somebody harvested it. And so on. Eating is a way to appreciate the interdependence of living systems. When done with awareness, eating can inspire gratitude for more than simply relieving of hunger.

To eat consciously (which generally means more slowly) with others is an act of communion. Food and eating together are core symbols in many religious traditions, and feasting has always been connected with celebrations of significance. To eat or drink together can be a way to seal a commitment. To share food with others is an expression of common necessity, as well as common potential.

The healthiest way to slow down speed eating is to start chewing, a long-forgotten activity in the repertoire of most modern people—adults as well as children. Walt Whitman once advised, "Drink your solids and chew your liquids." Chew your solids so well that they pass like liquids down your throat. Enjoy the sensation of liquids in your mouth. Chewing aids digestion because the saliva in the mouth initiates the breakdown of the complex carbohydrates in the food. Chewing can also be an outlet for stress, a training of your attention, and a means of strengthening your will. And that all adds up to increased patience and peace of mind.

Practice conscious undereating.

An Exercise in Good Nutrition

Think about your food consumption over the past two or three days. Does it reflect, essentially, the recommendations listed above? To which guidelines do you currently adhere regularly?

Which ones are more difficult for you to implement in your daily diet?

Choose one or two of the ten nutrition basics listed above that you will implement over the next few weeks. Don't burden yourself with trying to change everything at once. Write a contract with yourself stating what you will do, how long you will continue to do it, and what you will move on to next. For instance: "From now until the end of the month, I will eat at least one fresh fruit each day, and I will cut down on my use of table salt. Next month I will work on eating at least one serving of raw or lightly steamed vegetables every day."

Never eat more than you can lift.

MISS PIGGY

You may find it helpful to tape this contract onto your refrigerator or to share this exercise with a friend—someone who will remind you of your contract and encourage you to uphold it. Invite your friend to do the same.

18 Prevent Accidents

Commonsense safety is easily overlooked as an integral part of a personal wellness program. A person may exercise extreme caution about diet, yet be quite lax in attending to accident prevention.

Most accidents—both in the home and on the road—are easily preventable. No training is needed to put on a seat belt in the car or to buckle up young children in a car seat, but these simple gestures can save lives and dramatically decrease the chances of severe injury. It only takes a minute to ask your doctor or pharmacist to check your prescription and over-the-counter medications for possible adverse drug interactions. Over half of all prescriptions dispensed annually are taken incorrectly, and drug errors account for increasing numbers of deaths in hospitals and nursing homes. You already know many ways to prevent accidents, since most of it is basic good sense. Yet the complications and pressures of modern life may cause you to put these safety precautions low on your list of priorities. The memory jogger below encourages you to take action where you need it.

A Safety Survey

Jot down what you already know about each of the items listed below, or go over this list with your spouse, your children, or a friend, and use it as a basis for discussion.

What I know about safety and wellness with regard to:

* icy sidewalks and steps
* the use and maintenance of stairs and handrails
* slippery floors and movable area rugs
* wet, slippery surfaces, especially bathtubs
* children's access to prescription or over-the-counter drugs
* out-of-date prescriptions or over-the-counter drugs
* seat belts and air bags
* automobile tires, wiper blades, and antilock brakes
* car seats for children
* the speed limit

* driving or operating machinery while under the influence of alcohol or drugs
* escape plans in case of fire either at home or away
* overloaded, improperly fused electrical outlets
* poorly protected electrical wires
* the use of electrical equipment near water
* space heaters
* storing cleaning products, medicines, and poisons in homes where children live or visit
* using household cleaning products and pesticides that contain toxic substances
* emergency phone numbers
* the accessibility of first-aid supplies
* first-aid skills for choking, burns, shock, and so on
* protection from high sound and noise levels
* safe disposal of paints, paint thinners, gasoline, and oil
* children's toys

This list is not comprehensive. It is a place to start. We suggest that you add to it by taking a slow walk through and around your home, looking for safety hazards. Make notes about what needs to be done to make your home safe. Check off items that need attention soon. Prioritize your checked items. Take a calendar and assign, in order of priority, one or more items to this week and one or more items to each week thereafter, until all obvious potential hazards have been handled.

If you need more information about any of the items on your list, your public library is an excellent resource. Consult the front pages of your phone book, which should have a survival guide and a list of emergency phone numbers. Call your local Red Cross for information about safety training.

19 Keep Friendship Alive

The opposite of love is not hate, but indifference.

ANONYMOUS

People need people. And often they don't realize how great their need is until some moment of great joy or deep sorrow. At some point in your life you've probably experienced this yourself—wanting to share some great news with a friend or, perhaps during hard times, needing care and support from others.

Less obvious is the need for strong, positive day-to-day relationships. Just as children need to be physically touched, stroked, and held in order to develop normally, all people need emotional stroking for a healthy, well-balanced life. A "stroke" is any form of stimulation or recognition that arouses feelings. Strokes may be positive, such as smiles, hugs, and loving words, or negative, like brush-offs, cold stares, slaps, or reprimands. Whether they are positive or negative, "strokes" confirm that you exist and that you matter, and this validation is essential to human survival.

It's alarming to realize that if people don't get life-affirming strokes, they will seek them out in death-promoting ways rather than suffer the condition of being a nonentity. Many people use illnesses of body, mind, and spirit, both consciously and unconsciously, to get attention, touching, stimulation, and something to do.

When social contact is increased or loneliness reduced, the immune system seems to strengthen.

BLAIR JUSTICE,
Who Gets Sick

One of the healthiest things you can do for yourself is to cultivate vibrant friendships—the kind that will supply you with the genuine support everyone needs, friendships in which you can dare to reveal your feelings, act spontaneously, care, touch, and serve. Stimulating and supportive relationships with other human beings are tremendous blessings—to the body, the mind, and the spirit.

A twenty-year survey of adults in the U.S. reported that, regardless of health problems, people who participated in formal social networks of some type outlived those who did not. An affiliation with a social network was found to be the strongest predictor of longevity, even above age, sex, or health. "When people are counting on you, you have a reason to get up in the morning," one researcher said.

Keeping a Relationship Vibrant

Rich human relationships aren't sustained by accident. A good marriage lasts because it is renewed day after day after day. Healthy relationships of all kinds will last and deepen if, like other growing things, they are watered and fed, and even pruned on a regular basis. Making the sustenance and maintenance of friendships a part of everyday life is an invaluable enhancement of your wellness.

The following suggestions are from long-term friends and married partners for simple things you can do to nourish the relationships that are important to you and to guarantee a loving environment for yourself.

* RESPECT THE OTHER. Do this even when you disagree over issues. Approach your partner or a friend with the same deference that you would pay to some hero or heroine—a great person you admire. Be kind, be kind, be kind! Honor the differences between you, and avoid trying to control the other, even subtly, to suit

your ideas of who they are or how they should be. Encourage conversation that allows you both to share your goodness of spirit.

Love is giving someone the space to be who they are and who they are not.

WERNER ERHARD

* BE BRAND-NEW. Allow your friends and partners to be brand-new, too. Recognize another human being as a profound mystery that will never be solved. When you give up presuppositions about the way someone has "always been" you give the other a green light to change and grow. If you remember to stay new, you are more likely to continue the courtship—dress for dinner, bring flowers, or listen to the other's stories—with the same exhilaration and respect that you had when you first met.

* GIVE ATTENTION TO SMALL GESTURES. These will provide pleasure or happiness to your friend or partner. A hot cup of tea brought to their bed in the morning, remembering the other with a small gift or a card, a small compliment—these are the little touches that build great friendships.

* TAKE RISKS AND CONTINUE TO SHARE SOMETHING NEW. Keep growing in new ways yourself. Taking risks may be as simple as taking a seminar or class, reading books in areas that you generally don't explore, or traveling. Money needn't be an obstacle to experimentation and surprise. Honor your own dreams and

keep moving toward them—that builds your self-esteem and invites your friends and partners to do the same.

* RETAIN SOME RITUALS. Celebrate holidays or anniversaries of important occasions, or share your spiritual or religious practices with your friends and family. Honor your traditions and your roots.

* PRAY FOR EACH OTHER, AS WELL AS FOR OTHERS. Whatever form prayer takes in your life—a traditional religious form or a simple positive mental remembrance—it is a significant way to build your connections with others beyond mere physical contact.

* PUT ATTENTION INTO HONEST COMMUNICATION. Use empathic listening. Set aside times to periodically clear the air of any questions or resentments that may have been building between you. Read a book together about how to improve communications, or take a class or seminar on the subject. Give yourself permission to say no as well as yes to your friend, and you will be doing your friend a great favor in the long run.

See Chapter 20: Energize Your Communication—Become a Genuine Listener (page 142) to build up your communication skills.

Right now: Before reading any more in this book or starting another project, take five minutes to write a two- or three-line note of appreciation or thanks to someone you care about. Send it out in the next mail or e-mail.

20 Energize Your Communication—Become a Genuine Listener

Since most of us spend more than half of our time in communication as a listener, we should be experts at it by now. If you are, though, you are the rare exception. Most people listen passively, planning what they are going to say next, or they listen partially, jumping on the first few words they hear and extrapolating the rest. It is no wonder that communication often lacks energy and leaves people feeling drained, bored, joyless, angry, depressed, or helpless. In many conversations there is little actual communication. Poor listening is usually at the root of the problem.

Dynamic listening is more than simply hearing. And it is easy to confuse the two. Think about this distinction in the realm of music. You probably hear music of some sort almost every day—as background to a TV show or in the supermarket. Even if you are not consciously aware of hearing it, this music creates a mood. Rarely will you attend to the lyrics or dance to the rhythm of this kind of music. Now contrast this with your behavior at a concert, a symphony, or a dance. In these circumstances, your body is turned in the direction of the band or orchestra. You may experience an emotional rush as you allow the music in. You may involve your body with it, starting to sway or hum along, or to clap in time. When the music ends, you applaud or stand up and shout. Now you are listening dynamically.

Imagine giving that kind of attention to another human being—involving yourself actively in what they are saying. That's what it means to *listen* rather than merely to *hear*. Active listening forms the basis of strong interpersonal relationships. It encourages interaction with another, rather than the assumption of a passive role, like people usually take with doctors, teachers, and other experts. Active listening allows you to step inside the other person's shoes and see, hear, and feel the world from their perspective. With that advantage, miracles can happen between you and others.

Good listeners are made, not born. They are made by their willingness to observe the volumes that are spoken between the lines in ordinary conversation. Good listeners, for instance, "hear" a clenched fist or a look in the eye as much as they hear someone's words. Good listeners are patient and nonjudgmental. They acknowledge other people's views without immediately

I believe the greatest gift I can conceive of having from anyone is to be seen by them, heard by them, to be understood and touched by them. The greatest gift I can give is to see, hear, understand, and to touch another person. When this is done I feel contact has been made.

VIRGINIA SATIR

trying to correct them or help them. They assume that the speaker is *the expert* about themselves, and become a witness to the speaker's process of self-discovery. Good listeners aren't satisfied with partial data and don't presume to know what another person means. Good listeners ask questions to clarify meaning and paraphrase what they heard to be sure they understood what was said. Good listeners are an active presence. They look at you, smile, nod their head, or give other appropriate forms of nonverbal feedback. (Too much of this, however, can be a sign of trying to please without really listening.) A good listener can be a very good friend.

When you listen to me without interruption or
anything that feels like a judgement, you
allow me the time and space to get more in
touch with the many facets of me.
Thank you for never playing with my words,
getting a laugh or recognition at my expense.
When you allow me to revise or restructure what I
have said, I feel that you are truly committed to understanding me and what I'm about.
Thank you for not feeling that you necessarily
have to do something about what I share.
When you listen, I feel that you are listening

not only to my words but the feelings behind them.
Bless you for being you and thereby assisting me in my journey.

BENNETT KILPACK, MFCC

Barriers to Good Listening

The first step in any process of change is to become aware of what you are presently doing. You are probably not aware of the barriers you habitually put up to block good communication. Look over the list below and identify any barriers that you use.

* EVALUATING AND JUDGING. Are you so busy criticizing what the other person is saying that you don't hear them? There is nothing wrong with using discrimination, but it is more helpful to defer judgment until you fully understand what the other person is talking about.
* INTERRUPTING. When you don't allow the other person to complete a thought, you are not listening. Many people interrupt because they are impatient. If you find yourself losing the train of a conversation because the other is talking excessively, ask for a summary and then continue to listen.

* Jumping to conclusions. It is easy to mentally fill in the details of what another person is saying and then to assume you have understood them. People often take everything they hear personally, which is one of the main reasons for misunderstandings that lead to breakdowns in relationships. You can remedy that tendency by checking out your assumptions first.

* Selective listening. People tend to hear what they expect to hear, need to hear, or want to hear and block out the rest. For example, if you have been feeling a lack of confidence in yourself lately, you might hear everything that is said to you through a filter of "I'm no good." Or you might tune out everything that is critical, unpleasant, or negative because it is too threatening to hear right now. Keep in mind that everybody uses some form of selective listening. Get to know your form of selectivity and observe your tendency to block listening with it.

* Advising. You may think that you have to answer every question asked and solve every problem. Not true. The other person may simply be thinking aloud, asking rhetorical questions, or just looking for a supportive presence. In fact, as you share your advice, you may actually be disregarding what the other person is saying. Let others specifically ask for help or advice.

Otherwise, just listen and be there. One valuable way to encourage people to solve their own problems is to ask how they would advise a friend with a similar problem.

* LACK OF ATTENTION. Do you let your mind wander frequently in conversations, giving in to other external noises and distractions or to your own daydreams or plans? Often it is helpful to be up front about it—admit your temporary lack of attention to the person speaking; explain that you are sleepy, anxious, or whatever. If boredom is the problem, though, remember that the more involved you become in the conversation, the less boring it may be. Ask questions. Ask for examples. Summarize what you hear the other person saying. If all else fails, tell the other person honestly that you need to leave or get back to what you were doing. Good listening need not be a matter of silent endurance. Good listening is an active process.

Communication Theory: I know you believe you understand what you think I said. But I am not sure you realize that what you heard is not what I meant.

Toward Dynamic Listening

Consider which of the listening barriers cited above you practice. When do you most frequently use them? With whom? Why? Choose one listening block that you would like to chip away. Who would you like to practice better listening with? Under what circumstances?

Determine to watch yourself throughout your next interaction with that person, noticing how easily you fall into your habitual patterns of passivity or nonlistening and/or how well you implement your new active listening behavior. Make a tally sheet for yourself of how many times in that conversation you blocked communication, and how many times you broke through the block with active listening. Write about your experience to help clarify it for yourself.

Remember, you cannot change another person, but the quality of your relationship can be improved if you practice active listening.

21 Just Say No

The world-renowned family therapist Virginia Satir used to wear a medallion around her neck. The word *yes* was emblazoned on one side of the medallion, and on the other side, the word *no*. She often said that one of her primary tasks was to help her clients learn to say yes when they meant yes, and no when they meant no.

Those who work in the growing field of addiction recovery, especially recovery from codependence, emphasize the need for personal integrity—that is, honesty with yourself and others. Virginia Satir estimated that codependence afflicts over 90 percent of the U.S. population. "The disease of lost selfhood," as author Charles Whitfield, MD, calls codependency, is probably at the root of all other addictions. It results from focusing too much on what is outside of yourself and thereby depending on others to define what you think, how you feel, and what you do.

The High Cost of Yes

The advantage of telling the truth is you don't have remember what you said.

RITA MAE BROWN

While an attitude of openness to life is definitely health-promoting, saying yes to life means saying no a good deal of the time, too. People who are afraid of disapproval from others will say yes regardless of their true feelings to avoid rocking the boat. The question can range from the trivial ("Would you like a cup of coffee?") to the serious ("Can I stay at your apartment for a few weeks?"). When it comes to dealing with doctors or other caregivers, it is easy to fall into the trap of being a passive patient, afraid to say no to a suggested procedure, for instance, even though you may feel very ambivalent about it.

There is a high price to pay for such a lack of honesty in your personal relationships and in your dealings with professionals. Here's why:

* IT'S STRESSFUL. Holding in feelings of anger or frustration while smiling and saying yes causes unnecessary tension, and if you do this continually it may erupt in physical symptoms or emotional confusion and instability.

* IT'S CONFUSING. Other people will read the true message in your body language, tone of voice, or energy level. They will be unsure of what you are really saying and will question your trustworthiness.

* IT UNDERMINES YOURSELF. You erode your own self-esteem when you deny that you have insight, opinions, intuitions, and value judgments. By saying yes when you mean no, you give up your vote over what goes on in your own life. The more you deny yourself, the more you may feed feelings of low self-worth and set in motion the cycle of dishonesty/guilt/self-hatred/depression.

* IT DISEMPOWERS OTHERS. When you assume that other people will be upset or fall apart because you say no, you are assuming they do not have the strength to hold on to their own convictions. Genuine friendship or colleagueship cannot grow from such a weak foundation. Loneliness is often the result.

Learning to Say No

Admittedly, saying no is not easy if a lifetime of ambivalent yes-saying has preceded it. You may find that you are suddenly less popular with certain people (especially those who are afraid to think for themselves). Keep in mind that the practice of saying no does not imply being nasty, cold, or arrogant toward others. No is just no. It can still be said in a way that respects the other.

To practice saying no, you may want to start with matters of small consequence and work up to the bigger ones. Here are a variety of approaches:

* PRACTICE ON YOURSELF. Stand in front of a mirror and practice saying no in a variety of ways. Experiment with different phrases that feel natural to you: "No thank you, but thanks for asking." "Doing that would require more [time, work, money] than I'm willing to spend right now." "I've decided to cut back on my outside commitments in order to put more time into my [home life, schoolwork, relationship with my spouse]."

* WRITE OUT, IN SIMPLE SENTENCES, THE CLEAR NO MESSAGE THAT YOU MAY BE AFRAID TO DELIVER. Use this script when you need to call someone to say no or practice it before meeting someone in person. For

example: "I know that you need help on this project, and it was great to work on it with you last year, but I have other priorities at this time that require my attention, so I will be unable to assist you. Good luck in getting the volunteers you need, and please call me again for next year." Avoid apologizing. Practice your script until it sounds natural to you. The more often you speak in ways that are genuinely congruent with your own thoughts and feelings, the easier it will become.

* EXAMINE THE WAYS IN WHICH YOU CURRENTLY SPEND YOUR TIME AND ENERGY, including your diet and exercise programs. Determine which activities no longer support your wellbeing. Make a list of *No Mores* and post it where you will see it often. Check off one or two items you could most easily drop, and plan to get at them right away. Think back to the last time you wanted to say no but didn't. Recall, with as much detail as you can, your feelings about that situation. Forgive yourself for your lack of honesty, if that was the case. Decide whether you want to, if you can, remedy that situation by saying no now. In any case, reaffirm your intention to say no—as appropriate—in the future.

* REFLECT ON THE FOLLOWING INTEGRITY STATEMENTS. Such statements form the context for saying yes

and saying no in a way that honors yourself and others. Which of these statements are appealing to you? Which would you like to commit to? Which would you like to discuss with others? Write in your journal about the implications of each statement.

* I am willing to be more responsible for my own life in thought, speech, and action.
* I want to support others (in a manner that is kind, generous, and compassionate) in being more responsible for themselves.
* I wish to value interdependence in my life (we're all here together, humans and other creatures) and to live in harmony with that realization.
* I wish to honestly acknowledge both mistakes and successes, in myself and others, without judgment or overindulgence.
* I am willing to honor and respect my whole being: my body, my mind, my emotions, and my spirit.
* I want to remain open to feedback and flexible in my dealings with the environment, with myself, and with others.
* I value my word as a sacred pledge, to myself and to others, and wish to be more trustworthy and dependable, in small matters as well as in large ones.

* I wish to honor my dreams, goals, and ideals and to work toward bringing them into reality. I wish to honor the dreams, goals, and ideals of others, and to assist them (as appropriate) in bringing these into reality.
* I wish to ask for help and to allow people to help me as an expression of shared humanity, even if I'm feeling guilty, unworthy, or dependent.
* I wish to honor and trust my basic goodness.

You work that you may keep pace with the earth and the soul of the earth.

KAHLIL GIBRAN

22 Work Well

This poet's words come from an earlier time when people's work more directly supported their survival—they grew their own food and built their own homes with tools of their own fabrication. The principle applies no matter how you earn your living. There is an inherent value in doing work that keeps us all alive and well. In this sense there is no job that is ignoble.

But people tend to lose sight of the value of their work, getting so caught up in the details that they forget what they are doing or why they are doing it. Complaints are rife: too much pressure, too boring, the boss is impossible. Whatever the problem, the outcome is the same—job dissatisfaction leading to complete burnout and the feeling that you can't face another day on the job.

Most people spend a third or more of their lives in the workplace. It is very important, then, that work fully supports our wellbeing—physically, emotionally, relationally, intellectually, and spiritually. Your body can put up with abuse in the short run, but over years those abuses will take their toll.

A Few Steps toward Healthier Work

There are many ways to practice initiative and self-responsibility in the workplace without having to quit your job. You can make changes in your relationship to your job so it will satisfy you more deeply.

First, assess your relationship to your job in the light of the factors below.

* You like what you do even if you don't like all of the details of your job. Your job provides you with the opportunity to take on tasks, accomplish them, and feel good about yourself and about what you have created or produced.

* You have a sense of purpose in what you do. In other words, you have made the job important by the

way in which you define or view it. You appreciate yourself for working to support yourself and your family, even if your job is not ideal.

* YOU CAN DISTINGUISH BETWEEN THE JOB YOU DO AND WHO YOU ARE. You know that even if you don't accomplish all you set out to accomplish, or fail outright, or are unable to work or are unemployed, you are still a worthwhile human being.

* YOU SPEND TIME CULTIVATING OTHER INTERESTS and other aspects of yourself that your job doesn't include. You continue to learn, stretch, grow, and, especially, take small risks as ways to keep yourself flexible in body, mind, and soul.

* YOU PRACTICE SELF-RESPONSIBILITY, SAFETY, STRESS REDUCTION, AND HONEST COMMUNICATION as much as possible. You stand up as a person of clear integrity within your work environment.

* YOU FEEL GOOD WHEN YOU GET UP IN THE MORNING TO GO TO WORK. You experience general good health and rarely find it necessary to take a sick leave to cope with your job.

* YOUR SPOUSE AND CHILDREN APPRECIATE AND ENCOURAGE YOUR WORK. Your work allows you to spend quality time with your family.

Tell yourself the truth about your job and how it supports your wellbeing. Take a good long look at your job situation and the physical conditions in which you work. Make it a thorough look.

Imagine that you are a journalist doing a story on the healthiness of your workplace. Make a list of things that could be improved. Even though you may feel sure many things cannot be changed, list them anyway. Here are a few things to consider:

* sufficiency and type of lighting
* the quality of the air that circulates in your workplace
* access to the natural environment (Do you have a window in your area; can plants grow there?)
* the colors on the walls
* noise levels—of machinery or other workers
* telephone interruptions
* traffic patterns in your space
* the design and placement of furniture

Review your list and ask yourself whether these things serve your work and help you to work more efficiently and pleasantly, or if they undermine your health and your work.

Now examine the pace of your work. Does your job allow for periodic stretches? Do you have to spend hours sitting, or can you get up and walk around? (Many of us just settle for the inevitability of a work situation in which the needs of our bodies and minds will always be secondary to the demands of productivity. Changes in the work environment may require active steps on our part.) Who sets deadlines? Are they generally realistic? Are you expected to work overtime regularly or to take work home on weekends?

Look at the cultural norms in your office or work group. Is smoking or drinking encouraged? Are heavy lunches of high-fat food the usual fare? Is coffee the beverage that fuels work? Do other people support one another in exercise or working out in some way? Do you?

If there are difficult people with whom you have to interact, are you able to maintain your sense of self-worth despite their actions? If not, what internal messages do you give yourself when you leave these people? Are you self-critical, defensive, upset? What do you and your coworkers talk about when you are not working? Do these conversations create momentum for creative action and uplift or stimulate you, or are they full of gossip and generally depress, drain, or bore you?

That's a lot of investigating. Maybe you've opened up a few cans of worms that you hadn't wanted to touch. Summarize what you've discovered for yourself. Write a letter to yourself in which you describe the health of your current job situation.

Or give yourself a job-health quotient by assigning yourself a score between 1 and 100, where 100 indicates an ideal, high-health work environment and 1 means a work situation that is about to kill you.

See Chapter 3: Breathe for Life (page 32), Chapter 9: Stretch Yourself (page 70), Chapter 10: Loosen Up Your Belt and Everything Else (page 77) for breathing, stretching, and loosening up exercises that can be done at the workplace.

No matter how bad the situation may seem, realize that when you give up your voice in your own life, you become the victim of circumstances, and then you are lost. If you become an active participant in your life, you will maintain a sense of being in charge of your life. You do this by initiating changes, however small. Many times a small change is all it takes.

Make a distinction here: There are two levels at which you can make changes. The first is the behavioral level. At this level you will actually do something, or *not* do something, to effect a change in your environment. For example, you may have adjusted your chair to suit the height of your computer screen, but found that your legs are cramped. To make your working environment healthier, you put the monitor on a stand that raises it four inches. Now your chair can stay higher, giving your legs more room, and your neck doesn't have to be bent. Other small changes at this level can include negotiation with management for a healthier environment or a change of schedules to allow for flextime. You could also confer with your coworkers about instituting some changes. This can be more successful than trying to be a lone crusader.

The second level of making changes is attitudinal change. At this level you work within yourself, changing your perception, your degree of attachment, or your sense of purpose and intention with regard to your job. The proverbial cup appears half empty or half full depending upon the observer's attitude. It is up to you to define how your job gives meaning to your life and what overall purpose it serves. Meanings are in people, not in things. Recall Gibran's words, and choose the meaning your work has for the soul of the earth. Remember, it is not always possible to change what is, but it is always possible to change your relationship to it. The books listed in the resources section at the end of the book (page 213) will assist you in making this reorientation.

You may decide that the only solution to your problem is a job change. This is not something to be done hastily, even if it is economically feasible. Take time to review Chapter 5: Discover What You Already Know (page 46) and Chapter 8: Set Goals for the Changes You Want to Make (page 61) on goal setting. Then make a three-year plan that addresses your work life. What do you want to be doing three years from now? Where do you want to live? What income do you want to make? What do you want to learn? How do you want to grow?

23 Befriend the Earth

When the air in cities becomes so toxic that allergic and sensitive individuals must wear masks and eye shields, there is trouble afoot. When major segments of a population can no longer trust the quality of the local water and resort to using their own filtration systems or buying bottled water, it's time for some serious reevaluation of priorities.

In Greek mythology, the earth was seen as our mother and was called *Gaia*. The hypothesis that Gaia is a living entity, a single organism, was first suggested by Johannes Kepler hundreds of years ago. James Lovelock developed that concept further in *Gaia: A New Look at Life on Earth*. Observing that our planet has systems that closely regulate temperature, oxygen concentration, and at least twenty other variables, Lovelock reasoned that the earth is much more than a hunk of rock with different species of plants and animals living on it. Rather, he proposed that it is a whole system made up of many smaller systems, including humankind.

I begin to look at this earth as my home, and myself as part of everything here.

SUSAN GRIFFIN

There is no precise point at which the mind stops and the body starts. Similarly, there is no place where the individual stops and the environment starts, and vice versa. The nuclear accident at Chernobyl in the former Soviet Union affected the agriculture of the entire European continent. We are all interdependent. People no longer have the luxury of thinking of themselves as belonging to separate nations. Just as you cannot expect to find healthy fish in a polluted pond, you cannot expect to remain a healthy human being when you're breathing polluted air, eating devitalized food, and watching the earth being stripped of her resources. Wellness is an illusion if there is no commitment to the health of the whole planet.

Did You Know?

* If everyone in the U.S. recycled one-tenth of their used newspapers, it would save twenty-five million trees a year.

* Every ton of recycled office paper saves 380 gallons of oil.
* Recycling glass instead of manufacturing new glass from sand reduces related air pollution by 20 percent and water pollution by 50 percent.
* Americans recycled over two billion pounds of aluminum cans in 2000.
* If only 10 percent of the population purchased products with less plastic packaging 10 percent of the time, it would eliminate 144 million pounds of plastic from landfills and reduce industrial pollution caused by the manufacture of plastic packaging.

You Can Make a Difference

Contribute to a saner environment by examining your own lifestyle for waste. Start a family recycling program. Take the time to separate newspapers, glass, plastic, and metal items from your trash and send them to a local recycling center. Bring your own boxes or bags to the grocery store, buy in bulk, and buy foods and beverages in containers that can be recycled. Save and reuse mailing envelopes, boxes, packaging of all kinds, wrapping paper, aluminum foil, and so on. Contribute clothing, old furniture, and household items to charitable organizations that distribute them or prepare them for resale.

There are many other practical, everyday choices you can make that will contribute to your own health and support the earth at the same time.

* PLANT TREES. One million new urban trees would reduce CO_2 emissions in the U.S. by eighteen million tons and energy consumption by forty billion kilowatt-hours (worth ~$4 billion) annually.

* EAT LOWER ON THE FOOD CHAIN. The reliance on meat and meat products in the world's industrialized countries is upsetting the entire world economy, necessitating the destruction of rain forests and farmlands to support the grazing of beef cattle.

* CONSIDER REDUCING YOUR ENERGY "FOOTPRINT." Do this at home and in your workplace. Pay attention to how much energy you waste—lights left on, hot water running down the drain, excessive automobile use, and poor insulation with temperatures set too high in winter, too low in summer. Solar technology is growing in sophistication every year. You can install solar panels on your roof and reduce your draw from the power grid, sometimes even feeding power back

Nobody made a greater mistake than he [sic] who did nothing because he could only do a little.

EDMUND BURKE

into the grid during peak demand times and getting paid for it. Until we start thinking in terms of reducing our consumption and using alternative sources of energy, we will continue to live out of balance with the earth's self-regulating systems.

✻ REFLECT ON THE INTERDEPENDENCE OF ALL THINGS. Realize that everything you think or say or do has an effect—either for good or ill—on your state of health and ultimately on the health of Gaia. Share what you know.

Part IV
one step beyond

*

Part IV contains material of a more spiritual nature—areas that some may consider unconventional or uncomfortable. We believe these areas are integral to the study of wellness, touching upon essential human needs such as inner peace and a sense of meaning. Welcome to the pinnacle of your wellness journey, resplendent with new possibilities for your growth and healing.

Part IV introduces:
* using music to enhance your health
* cultivating silence for sanity
* spiritual dimensions of exercise
* creating a bigger context for health
* compassion for self and others

* mental visualization for healing and stress management
* risk taking
* learning to live in the here and now
* making a friend of death

24 Explore Healing Music and Sounds

Without music life would be a mistake.

NIETZSCHE

In the Greek myth of Orpheus, we find a powerful testimony to the power of music. Throughout his journey in the underworld, Orpheus played his lyre and sang. His music pacified the dark forces, bringing tears to the eyes of the gods and softening their hearts. Music stirs emotion. It is no wonder that music has been called the language of the soul. Music can soothe, energize, enervate, or fan passions. You've no doubt experienced the emotional effects of music at some point in your life—perhaps at a wedding, a graduation, or a funeral. In every culture, spiritual or religious ritual is accompanied by music, whether it involves the rousing drumbeat of a tribal dance, the mournful strains of a medieval requiem, the awakening call of a cantor, or the joyous chorus of hand-clapping gospel singers.

Music alters the body and the mind. Just as loud, harsh sounds can injure eardrums and set the nervous system on edge, so too can music and other gentle sounds, like the ocean or your own heartbeat, enhance deep relaxation, supply you with new energy, stimulate creativity, and even transport you into other states of consciousness. When used consciously, music is a form of healing. So when you are particularly stressed, feeling sick, or in pain (with a backache, arthritis, or a bothersome cold, for instance), try using a little music therapy on yourself. Plants grow better with certain types of music. Why shouldn't the same be true for you?

Lose Yourself in Music

The key to using music for healing is to allow yourself to become part of it. Many people listen to music critically, identifying the interactions of the various instruments or comparing the selection with other pieces. This is listening with the mind, whereas therapeutic listening is done with the whole body. Instead of paying attention with your head, concentrate from somewhere lower in your body. Imagine that your heart is listening; allow your abdomen to be filled with the music; let the music come in through your hands and feet; breathe it. Abandon yourself to the music, as if the sounds were waves or clouds that are carrying you away or supporting you.

Depending on the type of music you choose, this method of listening can be either deeply relaxing or highly energizing. Listening with this degree of openness will alter the frequency of your brain waves, your rate of respiration, and your blood pressure. Imagery can be stimulated, memories evoked, emotions released, and tension dissipated.

Are you ready to expand your sensory awareness and appreciation of music, or to experience the healing effects? Music and sound-healing expert Don Campbell, author of *The Mozart Effect,* suggests that you spend ten minutes of undivided listening time every day for five days.

On the first day, select a piece of your favorite music (something that does not have vocals). Then sit back or lie down and close your eyes. Breathe. Notice whatever you notice.

The second day, as you listen to the same piece, do some ordinary activity like washing dishes or opening your e-mail or writing out checks.

The third day, while you listen to the same piece, conduct the music, as if you are a famous maestro.

The fourth day, listen to the same piece of music while you eat a meal.

On the fifth day, relax the same way you did on day one. Notice the difference in your appreciation or any effect from day one.

Other Creative Uses of Sound for Wellness

* SING. Open your mouth, your eyes, your throat. Sing at the top of your lungs, or quietly hum under your breath. Use singing to lift your spirits and to breathe more fully. Chant or hum to get your energy vibrating. Repeat the same sound or phrase to relax you, raise your consciousness, or reprogram your body with a health-inspiring message.

* PLAY AN INSTRUMENT. Maybe it's time to dig out that old guitar, recorder, or drum, or to start taking lessons. For many people, playing music is both a form of releasing energy and relaxing, and a means of creative expression. Drums are particularly good for this and can be used without any instruction.

* LISTEN TO NATURAL SOUNDS. Hear the air move through your nostrils as you meditate. Use wind sounds in combination with visualization to help you clear certain conditions, like headaches or a sense of confusion. Use

water sounds for encouraging relaxation. The sounds of birds chirping are excellent for inspiring hope and joy. Be creative. Make up your own uses for natural sounds.

Build Your Repertoire

Perhaps you have plenty of musical favorites to choose from already, different selections to help you relax or to release built-up frustration. But if you don't, it may be time to start accumulating a music library of pieces that you can use for winding up or winding down. Many large music stores have a section of New Age instrumental music (also called Ambient or Space music) with a variety of interesting selections. Classical music also offers unending possibilities. See the following resources for some suggestions.

Contemporary Audio *

Anugama—*Shamanic Dream II*
One of the finest examples of healing music to date. Ideal for bodywork or movement.

Bruce BecVar—*Forever Blue Sky*
Bruce is a guitarist with a naturally commercial sound. His heartfelt guitar playing is augmented by orchestration

* Music selections for healing and wellness were compiled by Lloyd Barde, Backroads Distributors, Corte Madera, California. For a catalog or to order, call 800-767-4748.

and other effects that expand the sound of his music. Relaxed yet lively, this recording never gets old.

Patrick Bernhardt—*Solaris Universalis*
Patrick is a well-traveled Canadian artist with a heavenly voice and a gift for universally appealing music. This is his most popular release, with long tracks, multitracked Sanskrit mantras, and a spiritual feeling that is reminiscent of Enya's music.

Robert Haig Coxon—*The Silent Path*
Recommended to massage practitioners. The combining of gentle keyboards, Tibetan gongs, and orchestral instruments such as oboe and flute make for a deeply moving recording of peaceful music.

Jonathan Goldman—*The Lost Chord*
Deep chant and overtone. Wonderful music for meditation or deep listening, with a Tibetan influence. Based on the extensive training that Goldman has had with lamas from that part of the world.

Incantations—*Incantations*
This CD has probably accompanied numberless human

passages: births, deaths, healings, and celebrations. Keyboards, Middle Eastern doumbek rhythms, a jazz bassist/flute player, a percussionist, and two angelic singers join in this musical communion.

Deva Premal—*The Essence*
Beautiful chant recording, mostly sanskrit mantras, such as the "Gayitri Mantra." Deva Premal's magnificent voice and emotional expression set this apart from the field.

Raphael—*Music to Disappear In*
Neoclassical composing meets shamanic heart rhythms. Can be used for movement, deep listening, massage, and in other inspired settings.

Suzanne Sterling—*Bhakti*
This is chant/world music with original songs sung in English. Suzanne's superb voice, excellent production, and world music elements from the all-star supporting cast make this a highly popular vocal release.

Weave—*Cho Ku Rei*
This music is designed for Reiki healing and is equally effective for bodywork, meditation, simple relaxation, or

nighttime listening. Warm melodies, plenty of space between the musical passages, and an overall sense of wellbeing fill this recording.

Classical Audio

Bach—*The Six Brandenburg Concertos*
Evoke a wide variety of feelings.

Beethoven—*Symphony #6 in F, Opus 68 (Pastoral)*
Inspirational and soothing. For pure joy, listen to the famous "Ode to Joy" at the end of the *Ninth Symphony*.

Mozart—*Jupiter Symphony* and *Violin Concertos #3* and *#5*
Almost anything by Mozart is great, but these are particularly magical and joyful.

Tchaikovsky—*Swan Lake* ballet suite and *Sleeping Beauty* ballet suite. Dance with your heart.

25 Cultivate Sanity through Silence

When you need a quiet spot, it is rare to be able to find one free of noise from traffic, aircraft, office equipment, home appliances, TVs, or stereos. The

When real silence is dared, we can come very close to ourselves and to the deep center of the world.

JAMES CARROLL

noise pollution of modern society grows more strident every year. The background noise in urban environments has been increasing at the rate of about a decibel per year, yet people rarely notice the increased noise because they have learned to block it out. But the stress that it causes is not blocked. Besides the immediate danger of hearing loss due to long-term exposure to the extremely loud sounds at rock concerts and of certain machinery, high levels of noise increase stress and irritability.

Rest and quiet are necessary when you are healing from illness, as well as when you simply want to renew yourself from the forces of overstimulation that are a part of life in the fast lane. It is important to find or create a place where you can achieve some respite from noise, and to use that place for relaxation and healing, for creativity, and for contemplation or perhaps prayer. It is even more important to cultivate an interior silence—one that can be accessed even in the midst of the most distracting external noise. That's what meditation is all about.

Where or when can you experience silence? In a church, a library, in the middle of the night, in a wooded area, on a mountaintop, in your basement study. When was the last time you allowed yourself the gift of the sound of silence?

Fear of Silence

Many people experience great uneasiness when confronted with a lack of auditory input. Perhaps it is because silence forces them to think, to feel, to touch deep parts of themselves, to sense emptiness or meaninglessness. Learning to be comfortable with silence is really learning to be comfortable alone with yourself. It is one of the healthiest habits one can cultivate.

See Chapter 11: Find Your Center—Learn to Meditate (page 83) for more information on meditation.

Nature isn't silent. Listen to the sounds of a stream or a waterfall, the rush of the wind in the trees, the chirping of birds. Yet nature is one of the greatest teachers of what real silence is about. Learning to be comfortable in nature, alone, without other forms of stimulation like music, hobbies, or people to talk to, is part of the process of quieting your overactive mind and resting from the compulsiveness that drives life in these times.

Why not make a date with yourself in a quiet spot with nothing else to occupy you, and observe what happens.

Helpful Hints for a Quieter Home

At the very least, you can nourish yourself in a quieter home by eliminating some unnecessary noise. Here are some practical suggestions offered by the U.S. Environmental Protection Agency:

* Compare, if possible, the noise output of different brands of appliances before making your selection.
* Use caution in buying children's toys that can make intensive or explosive sounds.
* Use a foam pad under blenders and mixers.
* Use carpeting to absorb noise, especially in areas where there is a lot of foot traffic.
* Hang heavy drapes over the windows that are closest to outside noise sources.
* Put rubber or plastic treads on uncarpeted stairs. (They're safer, too.)
* Keep stereo and TV volumes down, and use headphones if others in the home want quiet.
* If you use a power mower or any other outdoor equipment, operate it at reasonable hours. The slower the engine setting, the quieter it will operate.

In the silence of the heart,
Your inner voice can be heard.
With the silence of the mind,
The heart can speak its truth.

26 Move Your Body and Move Your Soul

In Chapter 15: Move for the Health of It—Do Something Aerobic (page 109) we dealt at length with the connection between wellness and physical exercise. Now we invite you to move beyond the basics of exercising to consider movement in additional ways. When you think of exercise, you probably think solely in terms of heart rates, strength, and muscle tone. But because the body, mind, and soul are always connected, exercising also involves your mind and your spirit. How you move will affect how you think and feel about yourself, and vice versa. And both will affect how you view life and the world. Here's how it all connects in your exercise programs.

It is about 7:30 a.m. I have been up since before dawn. I have seen the world at its loveliest moment. I have run more than eight miles, made my body stronger, and enriched my soul. I will shave, have a hot shower that will seem exotic and sensual, eat, and be off to do what all of us do. The difference is—I own the day.

JOEL HENNING,
Holistic Running

Adhering to a regular exercise program is a statement of personal power. It says that you are in charge of your own life, that you have endurance, strength, flexibility, and determination. And these qualities will spill over into other domains of your life and work. You can apply your newfound endurance and flexibility to creative projects, to handling questions that arise in interpersonal relationships, to setting out plans for the fulfillment of your dreams, and even to addressing ways in which you can contribute to environmental concerns and world issues.

Regular exercise firms muscles, may help you shed pounds, and generally adds a healthy glow to your complexion. All of this can build a more positive self-concept. You like what you see and how you feel, and your sense of pride grows because of your commitment to yourself.

When your body is tense or contracted, it colors your mind's perception of the world. Problems seem more problematical, deadlines more deadly. But a moving body is less likely to hold tension. A good run or a vigorous swim, for instance, can be ideal ways to release a dangerous buildup of worry. As Joel Henning said in the previous quote, with exercise you can "own the day."

Exercise, like meditation, is a natural way of achieving an altered state of consciousness in which the rational and problem-oriented mind is temporarily put on hold. A deep sense of connectedness to all life and a sense of inner knowledge are potential benefits when exercise is done consciously.

Exercising can actually be a form of prayer—a thanksgiving for the privilege of having a body and for simply being alive. When the whole body is used in this way, spirit becomes united with flesh; spirituality is grounded in the things of everyday life. Yoga, the martial arts, and some forms of dance specifically use the exterior posture to foster inner spiritual attitudes, such as serenity, gratitude, courage, or one-pointedness. With practice, these exercise forms and the attitudes they foster will subtly start influencing all your daily activities. You learn to cook your food, drive to the office, and even do your income taxes with a heightened degree of focus, a greater thankfulness for life, and a sense of harmony even in the midst of doing things you don't particularly enjoy. Such conscious practice helps to build the matrix for understanding, accepting, and participating in the great process of life. And out of that alignment with life, purpose and meaning are created and revealed.

Health is a function of participation.

WERNER ERHARD

27 Create a Bigger Picture of Health

The "participation" that Erhard talks about is participation in relationships and participation in work that serves a vision or a context larger than your own personal survival. Your health and wellness are by-products of a life that is focused and ripe with meaning, full of generous engagement with others in the creation of a world that works for everybody. This insight is not new. Wise women and men throughout the ages have demonstrated an elegant unconcern for their own problems (physical or circumstantial) combined with a diligent commitment to the wellbeing of others. Such an orientation results in an observable radiance, a tangible strength of character and profound wisdom, as well as a remarkable ability for compassion even in the direst situations. Think of Mother Teresa. Think of the current Dalai Lama. Think of someone whom you admire.

People in Western industrialized nations have a great luxury of time and money to devote to personal health. But it may be beneficial to ask whether these populations are truly healthier and happier than other cultures as a result. Are we really well in body, mind, and spirit?

Obsession with health can be every bit as wasteful of your human potential as ignorance and carelessness can be. Focusing primarily on self-health may be endlessly fascinating, but it can also be tremendously isolating, exorbitantly expensive, and outrageously time consuming. Ultimately, overconcern for personal health keeps people imprisoned in a tiny cell, limiting the vast possibilities of creative expression and loving relationships that await them. The equation is really basic: in serving others, we serve ourselves. Or put another way: Creating a bigger vision and living in support of it, we put our personal concerns in perspective, and we are subsumed and fulfilled by a greater need, a greater possibility, a greater love.

Reaching Out

"People helping people" is a tried and true strategy for moving out of and beyond personal pain and suffering. You are not alone with whatever diseased condition you may be struggling with, even though it may often feel that way. People are typically ashamed of their weaknesses and vulnerability and fearful of more pain, all of which feeds their loneliness and isolation. Yet when someone opens a door by showing friendship or offering a hand of assistance, especially if they have walked the same path of pain or disease, that help can be tremendously beneficial, drawing you out of your closed world and inviting you into the larger world with others who share a common vulnerability.

Service to others in need can be a powerful remedy for your own pain or sense of alienation. There is relief in putting your own drama aside, for however long, in order to touch, with understanding, the life of another.

Few people can fail to generate a self-healing process when they become genuinely involved in healing others. . . . Selflessness is the greatest weapon in integrating and aiding the self.

THEODORE ISAAC RUBIN, MD

The best healers are often those who know illness intimately from their own experience.

Moving beyond Identification

To identify with something is to incorporate that thing (be it an object, a person, a job, a role, a thought, an action, a feeling, or a series of symptoms) within your definition of who you are. It's funny, but most people don't realize how closely their self-definition depends on a particular identification until that identification is challenged in some way. For example, people become identified with their jobs. When they lose their job, they lose their self-esteem.

When you are ill, illness tends to permeate your world, whether it is a simple cold or a chronic condition. Having asthma or having arthritis can easily become "being the woman with asthma" or "being the guy with arthritis." And you may come to identify yourself with that illness. You might use it, and abuse it, to judge yourself or to manipulate others. Some folks believe that illness or disease is some form of punishment. When they are sick, therefore, they feel guilty. They feel unloved and unlovable. They compound an already aggravated situation with negativity and self-judgment. To align with a bigger context of health means refusing to use illness or disease in this way.

Next time you find yourself "under the weather" or experiencing discomforting symptoms, watch the way your mind works. Illness can provide self-understanding, if you don't get stuck in it. Pay attention to what you identify with. Self-observation is the first and most crucial step in breaking unproductive habits about your health, like blaming or berating yourself, other people, or circumstances for your condition, or thinking that because you are ill you are somehow a failure.

Observation without self-judgment is the key. Seeing clearly what your mind is up to, especially when it is caught in a loop of negative feedback, will teach you to simply move forward, regardless of the mind's chatter.

Open to Prayer

Some people pray as a means of seeking comfort in difficult times. Others view prayer as a type of communion with a source of love or with the mystery that surrounds their lives. Because prayer, by its very definition, connects you with a higher power, or universal source, or deep innate wisdom, it can encourage a more expansive view of life. With prayer, the gift of health may be seen in a new perspective, which prizes health but does not assign it ultimate importance. The old adage, "If you've got your health, you've got everything," simply isn't true. There are values more transcendent and meaningful than personal health.

Prayer can also serve as a means of expressing your interrelatedness with others. Recent research indicates that people who are prayed for by others, even by people they don't know, receive benefit in the form of fewer complications in surgery and faster healing time. Science may question such studies and the efficacy of prayer for a long time. What is unquestionable, however, is what it does for you. When you direct care and attention outside yourself toward another person's wellbeing, when you unite yourself with others in the commonality of shared pain and shared humanity, there is no doubt that you are healthier for it.

Expanding Your Context

Here are a couple of ways to carry the bigger picture of health even further.

* Spend some quiet time, an hour if possible, in which you simply contemplate and/or write about the ideas presented above. For instance, what do you think about the statement, "Health is a function of participation"? What do you believe about the old adage, "If you've got your health, you've got everything"?
* Make a phone call to a friend or relative who is currently ill or dealing with some chronic condition. As you listen, silently support, love, and pray for the person without trying to solve any problems or without demanding anything for yourself. Just be there. Notice if this activity affects the way in which you view your own health concerns.

28 Heal with Compassion

Any program of self-change is bound to include some moments of discouragement. Disappointment and frustration are natural when the fantasy of immediate results is squashed, or the expectation of perfect discipline or consistency is not realized. It is common to start off with a great burst of energy and then slowly wind down. It is natural to set high initial goals and then have to reevaluate their feasibility. These are all normal turns in the

A great deal of chaos in the world occurs because people don't appreciate themselves. Having never developed sympathy or gentleness towards themselves, they cannot experience peace and harmony within themselves, and therefore what they project to others is also inharmonious and confused. . . . That kind of gentleness towards yourself and appreciation of yourself is very necessary. It provides the ground for helping yourself and others.

CHÖGYAM TRUNGPA, *Shambhala*

cycle of change. They happen to everyone. The challenge is to deal with these setbacks realistically without allowing them to build into self-hatred or cynicism. Compassion toward yourself and others is an integral part of the wellness journey.

There are times to be strict with yourself and times when you should ease up. Self-compassion is a way to handle disappointment and frustration and keep moving ahead with your efforts to change. As you practice self-compassion, which incorporates self-acceptance and self-forgiveness, you naturally learn greater compassion for the shortcomings of others. Such awareness reminds you to be flexible in your approach to life, contributing greatly to your overall wellness.

The High Price of "Should"

Valuable life energy is wasted in burdening yourself with guilt and blame. ("I should have done this." "I shouldn't have done that.") These "shoulds" are danger signs if they are accompanied by feelings of self-hatred. Approach them gently, with caution. You need to examine them to determine whether they are just hangovers from early training ("You should always smile") or whether they are self-imposed demands and unrealistic beliefs that have no basis in your current reality. ("I should do everything perfectly or not at all." "I should never let others see me as weak, or they will take advantage of me.")

Learn to observe yourself more honestly and to show compassion for any areas that are not meeting your expectations. This will help you stay well. Self-hatred can build up an internal rigidity that is stressful on your system. Your emotional energy becomes toxic and that negativity weakens your immune system. With compassion, you open yourself up again, letting energy flow more freely through your whole body, soothing your emotions and clearing your mind.

Many body-oriented therapies such as massage, Rolfing, and bioenergetics, are designed specifically to help release years of accumulated resentment and rigidity. Any effort to change will only be lasting and life supporting if it grows in a soil that has been nourished with compassion. Without the compulsiveness of shoulds, your journey to wellness can be a joyous adventure.

What Is Compassion?

The basis of compassion is an honest recognition of your own suffering and that of others. Suffering is part and parcel of being alive. We suffer when we stay attached to the past, afraid to embrace the future. We suffer when we make unrealistic demands on ourselves or others. We suffer when the people we love leave us. When you acknowledge that you are not perfect, and neither is anyone else, you develop a sense of compassion.

Compassion is not blindness or naivete, however. Just because you may experience compassion for a teenager who was arrested for shoplifting or for yourself for breaking a promise doesn't mean that you condone a theft or relieve yourself of the need to acknowledge your broken agreement and your responsibility to clear it up. With genuine compassion, we let go of the past; we release grievance, recrimination, and blame; and we attempt to reconcile. We do not assume, however, that this will necessarily change our circumstances or the attitudes and behaviors of those around us, though it could.

Showing yourself compassion does not mean becoming resigned to your problems. Compassion and resignation are two different things. Resignation is dry, passive, and lifeless. It is an attitude of defeat. Compassion is active and lively and requires your participation.

When you show yourself compassion, you willingly look below the surface of your behaviors or feelings. You find your true essence—your core of basic goodness that may have been temporarily obscured, but never diminished. When you see yourself (or others) honestly, compassion becomes much easier.

Compassion toward yourself or others can relax you physically and bring you peace of mind. Such harmony is the essence of healing. And with inner harmony, the situations and decisions that formerly seemed difficult or complex are suddenly simple, clear, and sometimes even easy.

The weight of the burden is the seriousness with which we take our separate and individual selves.

THOMAS MERTON

A Short Exercise in Compassion

1. Reflect on one or two ways in which you are hard on yourself. What do you blame yourself for? What do you feel bad or guilty about? What "mistake" in your recent past still burdens you with feelings of inadequacy or regret? For example:

I feel bad about overeating at almost every meal.

2. Identify any accompanying message(s) of self-hatred, personal judgments, or negative interpretations.
For example:

The messages I tell myself about my overeating are "I'm undisciplined, weak, and lazy."

3. Ask yourself whether you really want to change that behavior or problem. If the answer is yes, the most effective change will take place if you willingly adopt a nonjudgmental attitude toward yourself. Go on to Step 4. If your answer is no or maybe, read ahead anyway. It is important to accept yourself as much when you are ready to make a change as when you are not.

4. The key to compassion is honesty with yourself, about yourself. It is enhanced by a conscious intention to be compassionate with yourself and others. As you form your intention for compassion, keep in mind that compassion may not immediately arise as a feeling experience, so if you wait for your feelings to magically change, you might wait a long time. Compassion begins with a decision based in the reality of the human condition. And it is followed by the willingness and the effort to act on the basis of what you have decided. Quite simply, you make the intention to live in compassion with yourself or others, exert some effort in acting differently, just watch without judgment if you fall short of your goal, and then make the intention again.

Be patient. Your willingness to look at yourself and others in the world around you with open eyes, without defensiveness and denial, is a monumental step. Your intention to be compassionate will slowly change your mental programming and build your energy for spontaneous action. Enjoy your wellness journey.

29 Put Yourself in the Picture of Health

Humans are image-making creatures. As mentioned in Chapter 6: Watch Your Words—Avoid Illness Programming (page 52), even without knowing it, you are constantly making mental pictures. As someone gives you directions, you visualize the route. As you read about a place you have never visited, you envision what it must look like. Even though you may never have seen a gallstone or a tumor, the words suggest an image to your mind.

The interesting thing about images is that, somewhat like words, they create emotional states that affect brain chemistry, and brain chemistry will depress or strengthen every system in your body, including your immune system. It pays to know what types of imagery you are generating and how you can make that

The Serenity Prayer

God grant me the serenity
to accept the things I cannot
change,
The courage to change the
things I can,
And the wisdom to know the
difference.

Anonymous

imagery work for you. Visualization is a powerful tool for personal wellness.

In biofeedback training, for example, people learn to lower their blood pressure by imagining vapors rising from a sun-warmed lake. You can also learn to significantly raise the temperature of your hand by creating a mental picture of your hand being warmed by the sun or being immersed in warm water. Raising your hand temperature has certain health benefits. For instance, it is correlated with a decrease in headache pain.

What you see is what you get.

ANONYMOUS

Holistic cancer support services throughout the world suggest using visualizations along with either conventional or alternative therapies to induce remissions. Patients are routinely taught to combine periodic relaxation with visualizations of healthy, energetic cells fighting and destroying the weaker and disorganized cancer cells.

Visualization skills are taught to business executives to help them expand their creative thinking and to create mental pictures of the goals they want to accomplish. Athletes use visualization in conjunction with physical practice to refine their performance and to build self-confidence. In childbirth, visualization helps a woman remain relaxed and focused during labor.

Patients anticipating surgery use visualization to calm their fears and give them a sense of control over their internal states. Visualization is growing in popularity because it works.

Imagery Experience One—
Paint a Picture of Health for Yourself

Read this over and then guide yourself through it, or ask a friend to read it slowly to you as you follow the steps.

1. Take a moment to relax. Breathe deeply and let your body sink into your chair. Close your eyes. Now recall a time in your life when you felt great, when your body was as healthy as it could be. Imagine yourself doing something in that healthy state, such as taking a walk or dancing.

2. Notice how you are dressed in your mental picture. What does your complexion look like? How is your energy level? Use all your senses to absorb your picture of health. Notice the smile on your face. Breathe.

3. As you breathe, draw in that image so it deeply penetrates your body. Feel the energy and aliveness that you

have in the image. Hold your picture of health for a few minutes.

4. Now open your eyes. How do you feel?

This exercise is a good way to develop and actually feel the effects of healing imagery. As you become at ease with the process, you can use it to alleviate tension and discomfort associated with a variety of symptoms, such as nausea, headache, or muscle pain. The next imagery exercise will show you how.

Imagery Experience Two— Flip an Image for Symptom Relief

Your mental images may be keeping you stuck in pain, tension, and depression. But they can be "flipped over" to become healing images, and thus used to alleviate the same pain, tension, or depression.

Read over this whole exercise for yourself first, or ask a friend to read it to you as you follow the steps.

1. Focus on one problem area. Perhaps it is chronic tension in your right shoulder or the nausea you experience riding in a car or plane. (Even if you are not experiencing

any pain or tension now, you can use this exercise to prepare a healing image that will be available to you when you need it.) Note as many sensory aspects of this condition as you can. This will help you create a healing image. Ask yourself:

* Is there a picture associated with my problem or pain? (For instance, tight, knotted nautical ropes that represent tight muscles or a murky, stagnant pool that stands for nausea.)
* Is there a sound connected with my problem or pain? (For instance, a grinding or gurgling sound.)
* Is there a texture associated with it? (A sore throat, for instance, might feel like rough sandpaper; an upset stomach might feel slimy.)
* Is there a temperature associated with it? (A headache might feel hot; a broken arm might feel cold.)
* Is there a smell or taste associated with it?
* Is there a movement associated with it? (Churning, pounding, or stabbing?)

2. Now for the flipping part. What would the problem or pain look, feel, smell, sound, or taste like when it is alleviated or cured? Flip the image you have of your condition, substituting its opposite. For instance:

* Knotted ropes are slowly untied and loosely laid out on a deck.
* A stagnant pool is drained and filled with clear, sweet water.
* Sunlight penetrates the dark cloud of pain in your head.
* The sound of a bubbling brook replaces the pounding sound in your head.

3. Now relax. Take a few slow, deep breaths and recall the healing image you have just created. Use words if necessary to reinforce the image. For instance: "My head is filled with billowy, white clouds." Continue to rest for at least five or ten minutes (more if possible) as you hold the healing image in your mind's eye. As your mind wanders or if you are distracted by your pain, gently recall the healing image. Continue to use slow, gentle breathing to deepen your relaxation.

Don't be discouraged if you can't conjure up all the images we have suggested. Use the ones that are strongest for you. Be patient with yourself in anticipating results, but know that other people have used this exercise to great advantage. Give it a try.

Imagery Experience Three—
Make Your Dreams Come True

Look back to the beginning of this book where you designed a few specific goals for yourself as you began. Choose one of your primary goals and use imagery to form a picture of yourself with that goal already accomplished. For instance, if you are working to relieve backache, create, in your mind's eye, a picture of yourself moving around your house, or walking or dancing easily, without pain. You may enhance this approach by making a collage of pictures, all indicating the positive outcome of your desired goal. Posting this collage where you will see it often will inspire you to stay oriented toward your goal.

The first step . . . shall be to lose the way.

GALWAY KINNELL

30 Don't Play It Safe

Don't get the wrong idea! This is not a plea for foolhardiness, but rather a challenge to you to express more of your tremendous potential. To do so you need to cultivate stress up to a point, and you need to develop an appreciation for the lessons and potential growth that disease or problems can afford you.

Life is too close for comfort.

LEE LOZOWICK

You may have the impression that stress and disease are enemies and your job is to eliminate them from your life. But that is not true. Stress is necessary for life. Without it you'd be slithering on the ground instead of walking upright. Without it you'd be dead! Illness is a virtually unavoidable fact of life, and the sooner you accept it as a friend and teacher, the better off you will be.

We invite you to take risks—the kind that stretch you beyond your limited definitions of yourself and of what is possible. Life is a great adventure filled with impossible goals, which may seem beyond your grasp, but that you commit to all the same. To paraphrase Woody Allen, if you aren't making any mistakes, or if people aren't criticizing you, you probably aren't taking any risks. You probably aren't having any fun, and you certainly aren't living and growing to your fullest potential.

Health is a function of your participation in life. Those who play it too safe often end up lonely, isolated from others, or obsessed with their own health issues. Such attitudes limit one's world and weaken the immune system as well. How about it? When was the last time you took a risk? Did something uncharacteristic? Committed yourself to a great task?

Here are a few simple suggestions to help keep life "unsafe":

* AVOID THE WELL-BALANCED LIFE. A life that is perfectly balanced is safe, limited, homogenized, and boring. Any programs that promise complete harmony are sure setups for failure and disappointment.

* CULTIVATE CHAOS. Without chaos the possibility of serendipity is eliminated. Operate without your usual rules and schedules for a day or two, and refuse to let it be a problem. Let things break down and don't fix them; then deal with the consequences. Learn what happens.

* THINK STRESS. Build your inner strength by cultivating situations that tax your courage, discipline, and commitment. If you've got a problem that you think is big or important, give yourself a bigger problem by taking on a commitment to a task "bigger than you are." Now watch the first problem fall into place. And don't be fooled by thinking that it necessarily means you will have to work harder. Busy, committed people quickly learn to work smarter!

* RESIST COMFORT. Avoid the numbing effects of a "walking death" by maintaining an edge of discomfort for yourself. If you run for a sweater every time you're cold or

turn up the air conditioner every time you're hot, you're keeping yourself insulated in more ways than one. Appreciate unavoidable pain and use it to learn what stuff you're made of. Remedies that mask symptoms also mask the information that those symptoms might provide.

Be patient toward all that is unsolved in your heart and try to love the questions themselves . . . the point is to live everything. Live the questions now. Perhaps you will then gradually, without noticing it, live along some distant day into the answer.

Rainer Maria Rilke, *Letters to a Young Poet*

* "Pig out." The healthier your diet, the more important it is to indulge yourself, occasionally, with all the foods you think are "bad" for you (unless you are actually allergic to them).

* Put on some music, pump up the volume, and dance!

* Don't be nice. Be simple. Be straightforward. Be caring. Be daring. Be wild. Be silly. Be uncharacteristic. Be anything . . . but don't be N-I-C-E. Not all the time. You know what we mean. Yes, *nice* is a four-letter word.

* Apprentice yourself to greatness. There is nothing harder yet ultimately more satisfying than being stretched beyond the limited vision you have for yourself. Fraternize with people who provoke you to greatness, who make you uncomfortable, who ask more of you than you think is possible. Study what they have to teach you.

* Live your questions. It is a natural human phenomenon to find or see what we are looking for, and to overlook or miss what we haven't anticipated. Our

thoughts, and in this case our questions, will therefore mold our experience of reality. (For example, if you are fascinated by the nature and meaning of time, your questioning will motivate and direct you into situations where you will learn about time.) It is important to cultivate questions that are open-ended in order to live in an open-ended world. Otherwise we mold our world into black and white, and answer all questions with right or wrong, yes or no.

Right now: List some of the ways in which you currently play it safe in your life. Determine one rule you're willing to break, and do it.

The past is dead. The future is imaginary. Happiness can only be in the Eternal, Now Moment.

KEN KEYES

31 Be Here Now

The philosophy of taking one day at a time is a healthy one. When you live in either the past or the future, you miss what is going on right in front of your nose. When you are going through hard times, the habit of living essentially in the present, one day at a time, or even one hour at a time, can literally mean the difference between breakdown and sanity. Living in the moment can help you endure a seemingly unbearable situation and find meaning in the simplest things, even when circumstances appear hopeless.

Meanings constantly change because your life is constantly changing. The ring that you wore yesterday and treasured as a sign of eternal fidelity may be tarnishing in the back of your kitchen drawer tomorrow. Meanings are found in the present. Looking to the future for happiness or living on past glories is a sure setup for disappointment and a way to lose touch with what you most want and need to support your wellness today.

Truth has no special time of its own. Its hour is now . . . always.

ALBERT SCHWEITZER

Life is less satisfactory when it is lived only in a linear mode—constantly moving along a line that extends into the future, piling one experience upon another. It's a little like being a tourist in a great museum trying to see everything in a few hours. But fortunately we can learn to live in and savor the present moment. Poets and songwriters have struggled for ages to express this concept. "Today is the first day of the rest of your life" and other memorable quotes remind us to appreciate the present. Mystics and spiritual teachers have assured us of the same thing. Jesus said, "So, do not worry about tomorrow." Spiritual master Meher Baba continually reminded his friends: "Don't worry, be happy."

Ways to Stay Present

* Use your breath as a cue to remain present and receptive to all the sensations—sights, smells, sounds, textures, and tastes—and the many possibilities that each moment offers.
* Stop before every meal or each new task. Pray or reflect about what you are about to do so you don't miss it.
* Live one day at a time. Limit your worries to this day, at the very most. The quality of each day can always be upgraded by remembering how precious time is.
* Take time each day for silence and solitude. The simple practice of meditation or focused consciousness is the most powerful means of moving into the here and now and staying "here" more consistently.
* Exercise vigorously and regularly. Using your body physically can be a natural high—a means of altering your consciousness—and a powerful way to connect with the multisensory experience of life in the present moment.

Normally we do not so much look at things as overlook them.

ALAN WATTS

Right now: Look at your hands. Don't just glance at them; examine them at length. Discover something about your hands that you hadn't known or noticed before. Now touch your hands. Explore them and the many different ways they move. Feel them against your face. Smell them. Taste them. Sit and rest and look deeply at your hands as if they were your most precious friends. For the rest of this day, whenever you notice or think about your hands, let them remind you to breathe and relax into the present moment.

32 Make a Friend of Death

Recognizing mortality gives your life impetus unlike anything else. An awareness of your mortality urges you to use your time constructively to keep your priorities in order. From the perspective of your deathbed, things that are troubling you now might seem trivial and nonproblematical. Death is a fact of life; make death a friend. The Buddha, Siddhartha Guatama, started on his path to understanding and enlightenment when he first saw a dead body. It plunged him into deep reflection on the meaning of life.

Love the life you have; live sensuously and intensely. With death as your friend, you might live more consciously—caring for your health and wellbeing, honoring your body as the only one you've got. You might live more playfully—taking more risks and not taking yourself so seriously, playing life as a game! It is paradoxical that befriending death can increase your joy in life. You might live with more ecological awareness—realizing that your life and health, and that of your children, depends upon the life and health of this planetary body, Earth.

When you think about it, you are always "dying" in small ways every day, because you are always in the process of change. Change means saying good-bye to something in order to say hello to something else. Each good-bye is a little death. Baby teeth fall out, adult teeth move in. Skin cells die and are sloughed off as new skin replaces it. A new job means death to the previous one. Growing means death of old belief patterns.

Every moment you are being born to something new, as something old dies. Nothing lasts forever. As you become more aware of the death and rebirth in each moment, you reevaluate priorities. Treasure the transformative quality and possibility of each death and each birth. Celebrate the process of life instead of wasting valuable energy resisting change.

In some North American tribes, young men and women learn a death chant early in life. The chant is a particular repetition of words that reminds them of

There is an old story that Plato, in his deathbed, was asked by a friend if he would summarize his great life's work, the Dialogues, *in one statement. Plato, coming out of a reverie, looked at his friend and said, "Practice dying."*

STANLEY KELEMAN,
Living Your Dying

their destiny and helps them prepare for it throughout their lives. Whenever they are in danger, or ill, or frightened, they recall the death chant. It becomes a source of reassurance, something that builds personal strength.

Where to Begin

Look around you. Imagine that this is going to be the last day of your life. Don't just skim over the thought, let it sink in, as if you were an actor who had to face death in an important part. Think about how you would like to reorient your attitudes and your tasks to accommodate what you know is going to happen. Would you work differently? Would you relate to people differently? How do your big problems look from this perspective? Is there a person you want to contact to make peace with? Is there a letter that needs to be written? Have you made a will? Well, what are you waiting for? Do one thing to support your new view of your life.

Make a list of the things you fear about death. It might include the possibility of pain, being a burden to others, the hardship and sorrow that your death will be to your family, a sense of incompleteness, the feeling that you didn't do everything you intended to do with your life, or a sense of meaninglessness or that you never found your purpose.

Now ask yourself: How do these fears reflect upon the ways in which I live, or fail to live, my life now? What do my fears of death tell me about my real fears of life?

This is a valuable exercise to do with family members or friends. Talking about death allows people to share some of their deepest feelings. It is healthier to face your fears rather than to spend your precious life trying to hide from them.

Conclusion

Congratulations! You've reached the end of the book. By whatever means you arrived here—having gone step-by-step from beginning to end, or having skipped through, stopping only to address your most pressing needs—we hope that the small changes you've made have begun to make a difference in your life. We hope, too, that you are experiencing increased self-awareness and self-appreciation, that you have a sense of greater inner strength, and, above all, that you are living more well.

Wellness is a journey. We have started you off on the path to wellness. Evaluate your growth. Do you want to set new goals? If there were areas you passed over earlier, you could explore them now, or you could delve further into an area. Use the resources listed at the end of the book.

Whatever you do, don't stop now, because wellness is not a project to be completed and hung on the wall for display. It is an ongoing life process, a journey without end. So take advantage of the momentum you have now and continue on your way.

Be sure to check out the additional resources listed here and on our Web site: www.simplywell.org.

What Next?

Why not take a few moments now to summarize what you have learned about wellness so far. Using each of the unfinished sentences listed below, write as many responses to each one as you wish—the more the better.

* *Simply Well* has taught me. . . .
* After reading *Simply Well,* I am proud that I. . . .
* To support my wellness I want to. . . .
* To support my wellness I need to. . . .
* To support my wellness I will. . . .

Recommended Resources

*

Because of the volatile nature of the Web, we have not listed any web-based resources here, but refer you to our Web site: www.simplywell.org, which we keep current.

Here you can find access to such tools as the Wellness Inventory Online, links to most of the books that follow, and other resources specific to *Simply Well*, including updates and feedback from readers.

General Wellbeing

Capacchione, Lucia. *The Creative Journal: The Art of Finding Yourself.* Newcastle, 1989.

Chödron, Pema. *Start Where You Are: A Guide to Compassionate Living.* Shambhala, 1994.

Moss, Richard. *How Then Shall We Live?* Bantam, 1996.

Muller, W. *Sabbath: Finding Rest, Renewal, and Delight in Our Busy Lives.* Bantam, 2000.

Ryan, Regina Sara. *After Surgery, Illness and Trauma: 10 Practical Steps to Renewed Energy and Health.* Hohm, 2000.

Salzberg, Sharon, and Jon Kabat-Zinn. *Lovingkindness: The Revolutionary Art of Happiness.* Shambhala, 1997.

Travis, John, and Regina Sara Ryan. *Wellness Workbook.* Ten Speed Press, 1988.

Goal Setting

Covey, Steven. *The Seven Habits of Highly Effective People.* Simon and Schuster, 1990.
Koch, Richard. *The 80/20 Principle: The Secret to Success by Achieving More with Less.* Doubleday, 1999.
Levey, Joel, and Michele Levey. *Living in Balance: A Dynamic Approach for Creating Harmony and Wholeness in a Chaotic World.* Conari, 1998.

Breathing and Relaxation

Hendricks, Gay. *Conscious Breathing: Breathwork for Health, Stress Release, and Personal Mastery.* Bantam, 1995.
McKay, Matthew, Martha Davis, et al. *The Relaxation and Stress Reduction Workbook.* New Harbinger, 2000.

Meditation

Goldstein, Joseph. *Insight Meditation: The Practice of Freedom.* Shambhala, 1992.
LeShan, Lawrence. *How to Meditate: A Guide to Self-Discovery.* Little Brown, 1999.
Ram Dass. *Journey of Awakening: A Meditator's Guidebook.* Bantam, 1990.

Feelings and Emotions

Epstein, Mark. *Going to Pieces Without Falling Apart.* Broadway Books, 1999.
Goleman, Daniel. *Emotional Intelligence.* Bantam, 1996.

Simplifying Your Life

Andrews, Cecile. *The Circle of Simplicity: Return to the Good Life*. HarperCollins, 1998.

Dominguez, Joe, and Vicki Robbin. *Your Money or Your Life: Transforming Your Relationship with Money and Achieving Financial Independence*. Penguin, 1999.

Elgin, Duane. *Voluntary Simplicity: Toward a Way of Life That Is Outwardly Simple, Inwardly Rich*. Quill, 1993.

Luhrs, Janet. *The Simple Living Guide: A Sourcebook for Less Stressful, More Joyful Living*. Broadway Books, 1997.

Creativity and Health

Houston, Jean. *The Possible Human: A Course in Enhancing Your Physical, Mental, and Creative Abilities*. Tarcher, 1997.

Van Oeck, Roger. *A Whack on the Side of the Head: How You Can Be More Creative*. Warner Books, 1998.

Wellness and the Environment

Dadd-Redalia, Debra. *Home Safe Home: Protecting Yourself and Your Family from Everyday Toxics and Harmful Household Products in the Home*. Tarcher, 1997.

Johnson, Cait, and Maura D. Shaw. *Celebrating the Great Mother: A Handbook of Earth-Honoring Activities for Parents and Children*. Inner Traditions, 1995.

Lovelock, James. *Gaia: A New Look at Life on Earth*. Oxford University Press, 2000.

Robbins, John. *Diet for a New America: How Your Food Choices Affect Your Health, Happiness and the Future of Life on Earth*. Stillpoint, 1989.
Russell, Peter. *The Global Brain: The Evolution of Mass Mind from the Big Bang to the 21st Century*. Wiley, 2000.

Moving and Exercising

Anderson, Bob. *Stretching*. Shelter, 2000.
Hittleman, Richard. *Yoga: 28-Day Exercise Plan*. Workman, 1980.
Jordan, Peg. *The Fitness Instinct*. Rodale, 1999.
Lusk, Julie. *Desktop Yoga: The Anytime, Anywhere Relaxation Program*. Perigee, 1998.
Rosato, Frank. *Jogging and Walking for Health and Fitness*. Morton, 1995.
Yanker, Gary. *Walking Medicine*. McGraw Hill, 1990.

Massage and Touch

Downing, George. *The Massage Book*. Random House, 1998.
Kreiger, Dolores. *Therapeutic Touch: How to Use Your Hands to Help or Heal*. Prentice Hall, 1986.

Laughter and Lightness

Cousins, Norman. *Anatomy of an Illness*. Bantam, 1991.
Felible, Roma, and C. W. Metcalf. *Lighten Up: Survival Skills for People under Pressure*. Perseus, 1993.
Ornstein, Robert, and David Sobel. *Healthy Pleasures*. Perseus, 1990.

Eating and Nutrition

Balch, Phyllis, and James Balch. *Prescription for Nutritional Healing: A Practical A–Z Reference to Drug-Free Remedies Using Vitamins, Minerals, Herbs, and Food Supplements.* Avery, 2000.

Robertson, Laurel, Carol Flinders, and Brian Ruppenthal. The NEW *Laurel's Kitchen: A Handbook for Vegetarian Cooking and Nutrition.* Ten Speed Press, 1987.

Saltoon, Diana. *The Common Book of Consciousness: How to Take Charge of Your Lifestyle through Diet, Exercise and Meditation.* Celestial Arts, 1991.

Thomas, Lalitha. *10 Essential Foods.* Hohm, 1997.

Relationship Building

Hendricks, Gay. *Conscious Loving: The Journey to Co-Commitment.* Bantam, 1992.

Hendrix, Harvel. *Getting the Love You Want: A Guide for Couples.* HarperPerennial, 1990.

Lerner, Harriet. *The Dance of Intimacy: A Woman's Guide to Courageous Acts of Change in Key Relationships.* HarperCollins, 1990.

Ornish, Dean. *Love and Survival: The Scientific Basis for the Healing Power of Intimacy.* HarperCollins, 1998.

Listening and Communicating

Beattie, Melodie. *Codependent No More: How to Stop Controlling Others and Start Caring for Yourself.* Hazelden, 1996.

Bradshaw, John. *Healing the Shame That Binds You.* Health Communications, 1988.

Fanning, Patrick, Matthew McKay, and Martha Davis. *Message: The Communication Skills Book*. New Harbinger, 1995.
Fisher, Roger, et al. *Getting to Yes: Negotiating Agreement without Giving In*. Penguin, 1991.
Rosenberg, Marshall. *Nonviolent Communication: A Language of Compassion*. PuddleDancer, 1999.

Working and Playing

Bolles, Richard. *What Color Is Your Parachute? A Practical Guide for Job-Hunters and Career-Changers*. Ten Speed Press, revised annually.
McGee-Cooper, Anne. *You Don't Have to Go Home from Work Exhausted! A Program to Bring Joy, Energy, and Balance to Your Life*. Bantam, 1992.

Music and Sound

Bloomfield, Harold. "The Healing Silence." In *Healers on Healing*, R. Carlson and B. Shield, eds. Tarcher, 1989.
Campbell, Donald. *The Mozart Effect: Tapping the Power of Music to Heal the Body, Strengthen the Mind and Unlock the Creative Spirit*. Avon, 1997.

Imagery and Health

Achterberg, Jeanne. *Imagery in Healing*. Shambhala, 1985.
Borysenko, Joan. *Minding the Body, Mending the Mind*. Bantam, 1993.

Dossey, Larry. *Healing Words: The Power of Prayer and the Practice of Medicine.* Harper, 1997.
Gawain, Shakti. *Creative Visualization.* Nataraj Publishing, 1998.
Rossman, Martin. *Guided Imagery for Self-Healing: An Essential Resource for Anyone Seeking Wellness.* Kramer, 2000.
Simonton, Carl, Stephanie Matthews-Simonton, and James Creighton. *Getting Well Again.* Bantam, 1992.

Cultivating the Soul

Brennan, Barbara. *Light Emerging.* Bantam 1993.
Mitchell, Stephen. *Tao Te Ching: A New English Version.* HarperPerennial, 1992.
Moore, Thomas. *Original Self.* HarperCollins, 2000.
Walker, Brian Browne. *The I Ching or Book of Changes: A Guide to Life's Turning Points.* St. Martin's, 1993.

Death, Dying, and Being Present

Levine, Stephen. *A Year to Live: How to Live This Year As If It Were Your Last.* Three Rivers Press, 1998.
O'Reilly, Mary Rose. *Radical Presence: Teaching As Contemplative Practice.* Heinemann, 1998.
Ram Dass. *Still Here: Embracing Aging, Changing, and Dying.* Riverhead, 2000.
Ram Dass. *Be Here Now.* Crown, 1971.

Index

*

About The Authors

*

Regina Sara Ryan is a wellness consultant and managing editor for a small publishing company. She also serves as a graduate advisor in the fields of religious studies and human development at Prescott College, Prescott, Arizona. Regina is the coauthor of the *Wellness Workbook* (with John Travis) and the author of *No Child in My Life; Everywoman's Book of Common Wisdom; The Woman Awake: Feminine Wisdom for Spiritual Life;* and *After Surgery, Illness, or Trauma: 10 Practical Steps to Renewed Energy and Health.* She lives with her husband, Jere, in Prescott, Arizona.

John W. Travis, MD, MPH, founded the first wellness center (Wellness Resource Center) in 1975. He is the author of the *Wellness Inventory,* coauthor of the *Wellness Workbook* (with Regina Sara Ryan). He coauthored *Wellness for Helping Professionals* and *A Change of Heart: The Global Wellness Inventory* with his wife, Meryn Callander. Presently he is creating wellness tools for the Wellness Associates Web sites and several other Web sites such as www.theWellspring.com.

In 1993 John and Meryn gave birth at home to Siena, a curly-haired redhead. Since that time they have focused on the wellness of infants and young children, and are developing several books on this subject. Out of this work they cofounded the Alliance for Transforming the Lives of Children (www.aTLC.org).

Presently they live most of the year in East Gippsland, Victoria, Australia (Meryn's homeland) and spend extensive periods traveling across the U.S. in their 1971 Dodge camper promoting aTLC and visiting friends and colleagues.

Wellness Associates

Wellness Associates is a nonprofit foundation that grew out of the Wellness Resource Center, the first wellness center in the world, founded in Mill Valley, California, in 1975 by John W. Travis, MD, MPH. Dedicated to enhancing personal and planetary wellbeing, Wellness Associates supports people in developing the awareness and skills to move from domination and control to partnership and cooperation—a process we have labeled CultureMaking.

Besides our wellness books and questionnaires, we offer The Wellspring Online at www.theWellspring.com. The site begins with a list of common myths about children and growing up. These myths introduce the wide range of topics that ultimately determine our wellness in adult life. *The Wellspring Guide,* edited and produced by Meryn Callander, is a service for parents, caregivers, counselors, teachers, and children, offering in-depth synopses of books and other media for the heart, soul, and spirit of our children, our families, our future. In addition to the synopses, children's book reviews and links to supporting organizations and other publications are offered.

Write to Us

Your feedback and comments are valuable to us. Please share your thoughts and feelings about this book and mail them to:

Wellness Associates
Box 8422S
Asheville, NC 28814

Or e-mail to:

info@simplywell.org

Dear Regina and John:

Special Offer

If you enjoyed this book and want to learn more about wellness, you can order the *Wellness Workbook* from Wellness Associates for $19.95 postpaid (to U.S. addresses). If you fill out the feedback page on the opposite side of this order form, we'll include—at no extra charge—a copy of the Wellness Inventory (you can also order the Wellness Inventory separately).

Please send me:
_____ copies of the *Wellness Workbook* at $19.95
_____ copies of the *Wellness Inventory* at $2.95 each
_____ copies of *Wellness for Helping Professionals* at $49.50 each
_____ more information on the above titles

I am enclosing payment by ____check or money order ____VISA or Mastercard

Name as it appears on card____
VISA or Mastercard # ______________________________ Expiration date__________
Signature____

Ship to address:____
City______________________________________State__________Zip__________

Send your order to:
Wellness Associates
Box 8422S
Asheville, NC 28814

Or visit:
www.TheWellspring.com